The Infertility Treadmill

STUDIES IN SOCIAL MEDICINE
Allan M. Brandt and Larry R. Churchill, editors

KAREY HARWOOD

The Infertility Treadmill

FEMINIST ETHICS,
PERSONAL CHOICE,
AND THE USE OF
REPRODUCTIVE
TECHNOLOGIES

THE UNIVERSITY OF NORTH CAROLINA PRESS
CHAPEL HILL

© 2007 Karey Harwood
All rights reserved
Manufactured in the United States of America

Designed by Jacquline Johnson
Set in Ehrhardt MT
by Keystone Typesetting, Inc.

This book was published with the assistance of the Anniversary Endowment Fund of the University of North Carolina Press.

The paper in this book meets the guidelines for permanence and durability of the Committee on Production Guidelines for Book Longevity of the Council on Library Resources.

Library of Congress Cataloging-in-Publication Data
Harwood, Karey.
The infertility treadmill : feminist ethics, personal choice, and the use of reproductive technologies / Karey Harwood
p. cm. — (Studies in social medicine.)
Includes bibliographical references and index.
ISBN-13: 978-0-8078-3157-1 (cloth : alk. paper)
ISBN-13: 978-0-8078-5847-9 (pbk. : alk. paper)
1. Human reproductive technology—Social aspects.
2. Feminist ethics. I. Title.
RG133.5.H384 2007
618.1'7806—dc22   2007020208

cloth   11 10 09 08 07   5 4 3 2 1

paper   11 10 09 08 07   5 4 3 2 1

TO MY SONS, JAMES, WESLEY, AND ANDREW

Contents

Acknowledgments

I am very grateful to the leaders and members of RESOLVE of Georgia who allowed me to join their monthly meetings and learn from their struggles with infertility. This book would not have been possible without the openness of individuals who were willing to share their stories with each other and with me.

I was fortunate to receive a 2001 Woodrow Wilson Dissertation Grant in women's health that supported my research and the transcription of interviews. I also benefited from the wise counsel of Elizabeth Bounds, Jon Gunnemann, Nancy Eiesland, Timothy Jackson, and Steve Tipton, all of Emory University. Their insights into this project and its methodology enabled me to analyze a wealth of qualitative data with both care and conviction.

Several colleagues, including Marie Marquardt, Barbara McClure, Brad Schmeling, and Melissa Snarr, read and commented on early stages of the book. I remain indebted to their clear thinking and helpful suggestions.

As an assistant professor at North Carolina State University, I have enjoyed a great deal of support during the final stages of writing this book. I thank Michael Pendlebury and Jason Bivins for their encouragement. I also thank Ann Rives for her excellent help in preparing the manuscript and index.

From the beginning of the publication process, I have had the expert guidance of Sian Hunter, senior editor at the University of North Carolina Press. I surely would not have made it this far without her careful reading and attention to detail. I am deeply grateful to Paula Wald, associate managing editor at UNC Press; Ellen Goldlust-Gingrich, who copyedited this volume with great care; and Ashley Mason for proofreading.

In addition, I owe an enormous debt of gratitude to my family. My parents, Phyllis and David Harwood, provided crucial hours of child care for my three sons as well as significant intellectual contributions to many of the chapters.

My in-laws, Martha and Frank Wood, have similarly supported my efforts in ways large and small.

This project began when my oldest son was in preschool. He and his two younger brothers have literally grown up with this book. I thank them for their patience and for reminding me of all the goods of family life. Finally, none of the work would have been possible without the love and commitment of my husband, Swain Wood.

The Infertility Treadmill

Work, Family, and Reproductive Technologies

Sarah was thirty-five years old when she discovered she was infertile. A critical-care nurse, Sarah had married her husband in her early thirties, and they had intended to spend a couple of years settling into their marriage before embarking on parenthood. When they decided to start actively trying to conceive, they were not in any hurry. Sarah's husband traveled a lot for work, so she was not concerned when she did not become pregnant right away. But after a year had passed, Sarah started to worry. She talked to her regular gynecologist, and she and her husband began a regimen of tests to discover the source of the problem, starting with the most basic: the "postcoital" and semen analysis. To her gynecologist's thinking, everything seemed more or less normal, and he told Sarah and her husband that it was probably just a matter of timing: timing intercourse to coincide better with ovulation. However, Sarah's age was a concern. At the limits of his expertise, Sarah's gynecologist advised them to consult an infertility specialist and to "go straight to IVF," especially if they hoped to have more than one child.[1]

The specialist, through more sophisticated testing, quickly ascertained that Sarah's level of follicle-stimulating hormone (FSH) was elevated—not by a lot, but any level above normal is problematic for a woman's fertility, as FSH directly affects the availability of a mature egg each month. With this news, Sarah realized that she had wasted precious time with her regular gynecologist, not pursuing the problem aggressively enough. The specialist also informed her that her chances of becoming pregnant and carrying the pregnancy to term had plummeted to 6–8 percent. Though in retrospect Sarah claims that doing so was spectacularly ill advised, she and her husband decided to try to become pregnant via in vitro fertilization (IVF) using her own eggs—if any eggs could be retrieved. Their insurance would cover the procedure, which otherwise would have cost them between fifteen and eighteen thousand dollars out of pocket, so they decided to give it a try to avoid being later troubled by regret.

To their amazement, the powerful drugs used to stimulate a woman's ovaries in an IVF procedure enabled Sarah's doctor to retrieve a couple of healthy eggs, both of which were fertilized in the lab with her husband's sperm. The embryos were implanted in Sarah's uterus and she was, to her astonishment, pregnant. Sadly, the pregnancy lasted only nine weeks, at which time she miscarried, losing not only the pregnancy but also her hope of having a biologically related child. She spent months depressed, questioning her faith in God, questioning her judgment and that of her doctors, questioning the ethics of trying a procedure because an insurance company would foot the bill, and most of all questioning the unbelievable odds that she would become pregnant but lose the pregnancy so quickly.

After emerging from their grief, Sarah and her husband seriously considered using an egg donor, an option that the infertility specialist had presented early on as offering them the best chance of success. Then, for various reasons, complex and carefully thought through, they decided to adopt two little boys. Now an enthusiastic advocate for adoption, Sarah casts a critical eye on the infertility industry and those who endorse it wholesale.

Sarah's story is in many ways typical of the women that I got to know through my research with RESOLVE, an organization that supports people facing infertility: the belated discovery of a fertility problem, the jump to high-tech treatment in a race against time, and the desperate desire to try all available procedures to avoid regret. This book explains my research, what I learned from a year of listening to the stories of people struggling with infertility, and what can be said on behalf of the infertility industry, by which I mean the constellation of specialized fertility clinics and pharmaceutical companies that seek to fulfill people's need to become pregnant.

However, before I heard Sarah's story and the stories of so many others, I had my own reasons for investigating assisted reproductive technologies (ART). I did not wait to have children and struggled to balance parenthood with graduate school, and I wondered whether ART was helping women to "have it all"—both a career and, in good time, a family. Did ART implicitly promise to extend women's fertility? I also wondered whether this option had a darker side that did not receive the critical attention that it deserved both from ethicists and from policymakers who might be in a position to regulate the burgeoning infertility industry.

Motivation for the Project

One small news story during the summer of 2000 crystallized many of the concerns that had originally engendered my interest in ART. Dr. Roger Gosden, a scientist then at McGill University in Montreal, Canada, announced that he was in the preliminary stages of creating a "career" birth control pill. Gosden saw the benefits of the career pill as twofold: it would be highly effective birth control, and it would improve fertility for women between ages thirty-five and fifty. The pill would shut down a woman's egg supply during her teens and twenties, when many women, particularly those in the middle class, pursue education and career, but would preserve the ovaries for use when the woman reached her thirties, forties, and fifties. Essentially, the career pill would delay menopause and allow women to hoard their eggs until later years. According to the article, "Gosden said the new contraceptive could meet the needs of a changing society. . . . The pill would suit the needs of young professionals, either in higher education or starting their careers, who want to start their families later. It would give women control over their fertility during their younger years while extending their potential years for motherhood past the norm."[2]

What concerned me about the theoretical possibility of a career pill, which I viewed as at least symbolically connected to other reproductive technologies,[3] was that it asked women's bodies to accommodate the arbitrary structures of a "changing society," rather than the other way around. Like most methods of birth control, the career pill would have women assume all the health risks and endure all of the bodily discomforts while men assumed neither. But even more pronounced in the case of the career pill would be the explicit expectation that bodily norms would be altered to fit into society's age-graded educational and employment structures. It would offer contraception with a particular social purpose. The name "career pill" also seemed to suggest that the ability to postpone childbearing would be marketed to professional women as a self-evident good.

Why do these things cause concern? As a feminist and someone who came of age during the 1980s, I appreciate the fact that more women than ever enjoy careers that benefit them personally as well as contribute to the wider society, at least in countries such as the United States. These accomplishments are not to be taken for granted: they have in large part resulted from the women's movement's hard-won battles. American women of my generation enjoy a certain luxury in the decisions we make about work and family that women of prior generations could only imagine. Yet even granting the unique historical position of contemporary American women of childbearing age, I still question the implications of a *career* pill: why, for example, after women's significant gains in the workplace and the professions, do we still conceptualize work and family as an either/or dilemma that is fundamentally women's burden to resolve?[4] Evidently, women either forgo educational and employment opportunities to have children or forgo—or delay—having children to pursue education and employment outside the home. Why, we could ask, do the practices and policies of American workplaces and educational institutions not more adequately accommodate the reality of childbearing and child rearing as a fact of human existence—for example, through high-quality and accessible child care, paid parenting leave for mothers and fathers, and/or part-time work for one or both parents with benefits and without penalty?

The career pill seemed to me potentially to be coated in the appealing language of individual choice, freedom, and reproductive control but in reality to provide a convenient means of avoiding the hard work of restructuring society to be more just. As feminist economist Nancy Folbre argues, raising children is not simply another form of personal satisfaction that people freely choose, like having a pet. Rather, the flourishing of an entire society depends on the willingness—especially that of women, who still do the majority of care work—to bear and rear children. In return for that investment of time and energy, no matter how freely given, society owes parents support.[5] Because the career pill places burdens that ought to be borne by society as a whole back onto the bodies of individual women, it raises issues of social justice, particularly gender justice. The career pill crystallizes in a stark way some of the pressures American women face in trying to combine aspirations that most men take for granted: the desire to have a family and the desire to pursue some kind of personally rewarding, paid employment.

When I began the research for this book, I saw a strong symbolic connection between the career pill and ART. Both the career pill (which remains a futuristic dream) and ART (which is a medical commonplace across the country) can be interpreted as biotechnological responses to a cultural trend toward delayed childbearing. More obviously, the theoretical career pill constitutes a response to delayed childbearing. Researchers clearly believe consumer demand does or will exist for a contraceptive that enables women to postpone and preserve their fertility; meeting this need is one of the career pill's intrinsic goals. However, ART can also be interpreted as a response to delayed childbearing if one considers the relationship between increased delayed childbearing (at least among professional-class women) and increased ART use (at least among white middle-class women) as more than coincidental. Many causes of infertility are, of course, not age related, just as there are many reasons why more people than ever before seek out medical treatment for their infertility, including the simple fact that medical treatment for infertility is far more effective now than in the past. Yet several studies have demonstrated a connection between age-related infertility and the dramatic increase in ART use.[6] Some women clearly turn to ART to solve the problem of infertility—as they might some day use the career pill to prevent the problem of infertility—because of the effects of intentionally delayed childbearing.[7]

Less clear is whether women intentionally choose to delay childbearing because they know of the availability of ART. In a 2001 survey by the National Parenting Association, almost 90 percent of women between the ages of twenty-eight and forty who participated said they believed ART would make it possible for them to get pregnant into their forties.[8] A bold advertising campaign launched in 2001 by the American Society of Reproductive Medicine would also seem to suggest that many women delay childbearing because of their perception that ART affords them more time to have children: The large ads, placed on the sides of city buses, sought to warn women about the limitations of assisted reproduction and to educate them about the importance of age as a factor in infertility. They featured a picture of an upside-down baby bottle in the shape of an hourglass and cautioned, "Advancing Age Decreases Your Ability to Have Children."[9]

To the extent that ART may offer women a way to beat the biological clock and/or a promise of resolution to the persistent conflict between work and family, it may function as the current technological method for adapting biology to the structures of society—the cultural reality that makes dreaming up a career pill even possible. If this is the case, then it seems fitting to ask whether ART in fact offers an effective way out of the time trap and if so, for how many women? Does it benefit mainly women of a certain class and race? How does its use affect whether the biological differences between men and women are transformed into social inequalities? In short, how does ART affect the cause of gender justice?

In addition to these questions, which are rooted in a concern for fairness, I also brought some broader concerns to this project: How does the availability of ART affect the ways women and men understand what it means to have a family? Is the use of ART a healthy development for the physical well-being of women, their children, and future generations? And, most basically, what ends or goals does ART serve, and how should they be evaluated?

Overview of the Book and Reflection on Method

As the infertility industry grows to meet increased demand for its services and becomes more rationalized and accepted, the ethical significance of the decision to use ART can seem less salient: What was once seen as a morally radical option is now seen as one medical choice among many in a lifetime—simply one manifestation of a well-defended procreative liberty. However, when the individual decision to use ART is viewed not only as an exercise of autonomous choice but also as a social phenomenon taking place within a wider context of important institutional and structural constraints and incentives, then the ethical significance of ART becomes more compelling. It then becomes important to ask how individual beliefs coexist with and are influenced by social and cultural forces.

When I began this project, I set out to identify and evaluate the various factors that influence the use of ART, with a special concern for the role of work/family conflicts and the effects of delayed childbearing. Rather than relying on existing statistics and surveys, I chose to do my own qualitative research to test my concerns and assumptions against a social world.[10] The reasons for this methodological choice are multifaceted and are important for understanding the book's development.

I chose to do qualitative research, by which I mean gathering nonquantifiable empirical data through participant observation and interviewing, primarily because of my commitment to honor the lived experience of people who use ART while bringing some critical questions to bear on that use. I wanted to engage in ethical argumentation that was both empathetic and analytic. I also chose to do qualitative research because I believe in the value of the case study and in the power of example—that I could learn a great deal about the ethical questions at stake in using ART by listening carefully to people who use it and that the knowledge I gained from these observations would be potentially generalizable.

I also believed that doing sustained, respectful analysis of a group of people would provide more insight into the social influences on decision making than would any other kind of research. As Bent Flyvbjerg contends in his defense of the case study as a research method, "If one thus assumes that the goal of the researcher's work is to understand and learn about the phenomena being studied, then research is simply a form of learning. . . . [T]he most advanced form of understanding is achieved when researchers place themselves within the context being studied. Only in this way can researchers understand the viewpoints and the behavior which characterize social actors."[11] Even more to the point, anthropologist Lila Abu-Lughod argues that paying attention to particularity—the everyday language and experiences of individual people—is the best way to gain insight into the "larger forces" of society "because these forces are only embodied in the actions of individuals living in time and place."[12]

Thus, I decided to meet and talk with people facing the decision to use ART and to study RESOLVE, a prominent organization that supports people in their struggle with infertility. I will say more about how and why I came to choose this particular organization, as well as the precise research methods used, in chapter 2 and appendix A. I began my field research with an open mind about what I would find and a willingness to let the voices of people experiencing infertility take my project in new directions. I sought not to confirm existing theories but to challenge and refine them with details from and interpretations of a social world.

I found that the work/family issue constitutes only part of the picture. The rich, powerful stories I heard from people who attended RESOLVE meetings gradually drew my attention away from my initial focus on social structures and academic debates about sexual inequality in the workplace and family and toward more personal, existential questions of human beings facing insurmountable limits. ART played a crucial, if very costly and painful, role in many individuals' journeys to come to terms with their infertility, regardless of whether they succeeded in having a biological child. Yet even as my appreciation for individuals' struggles with infertility grew, I noticed gaping silences in the public conversations I observed. In the name of respecting difference and choice, RESOLVE participants offered very little critical comment about the infertility industry or any of the social forces that compel people to use ART, especially the force of consumerism. Many people talked about getting stuck on the "treadmill of infertility," a metaphor commonly used to describe what trying infertility treatments feels like, but very few people questioned how they could have avoided the ordeal. In other words, many of my concerns about social structures and social justice remain relevant, although in some new ways.

During the time I spent working on this volume, several other books have been published on the subjects of assisted reproduction and work/family conflicts, most notably Sylvia Ann Hewlett's *Creating a Life: Professional Women and the Quest for Children* (2002). This book generated some media controversy by recommending that young women be "intentional" about the planning of their personal lives, including the timing of marriage and children, to avoid missing the opportunity to have children while pursuing a professional career. Hewlett advises young women not to delay childbearing and not to rely on the "empty promise" of reproductive technologies, which, she argues, are far less effective in reality than media coverage of celebrity success stories would suggest. She also cites mounting evidence linking reproductive technologies with long-term health risks such as ovarian cancer.

Hewlett has been criticized for, among other things, placing too much emphasis on individual planning and choice, as if the problems of work and family conflicts could be solved by being savvy and strategic, by finding an occupation where "you can bend the rules," and by working hard enough "to deserve having those rules bent for you."[13] Although Hewlett proposes several government and private-sector initiatives that would help lessen the time crunch for all working women,[14] she tends to overestimate the power of individual choice and planning in solving social structural problems. More precisely, Hewlett seems less interested in truly solving these problems than in advising ambitious and entrepreneurial young women about how to navigate shrewdly around these obstacles.[15] However, the desire for a more just society that would benefit all women seems to motivate her entire project.

My book is similarly driven by a concern for social justice, as indicated by my comparison of the career pill and ART, but its primary goal and ultimate contribution is not to propose specific solutions to the work / family problem. This book seeks first and foremost to offer an interpretation of the ethical significance of the increasing use of ART by bringing a particular set of normative or evaluative lenses to bear on a particular set of descriptive data. This endeavor is fundamentally an act of *phronesis*, or what H. R. Niebuhr called "responsible ethics,"[16] which is best described as a dialectical engagement between concrete experiences and abstract ideas in which the observation of reality is focused and directed by preexisting normative values and agendas while the discernment of important ethical issues is, in turn, enlarged and refined by the observation of a particular reality. One learns and is changed by one's observations, even as what one sees is itself a function of one's beliefs and prior commitments.

In chapter 1, I set forth my theoretical starting points and normative lenses, formed primarily by feminist and Christian ethics, and elaborate the reasons why I think ART might negatively affect gender justice and human flourishing. Over the course of the next several chapters, I describe one particular community's encounter with the options available for dealing with infertility, drawing on a year of field research with RESOLVE. Here I sketch what emerged as the group's ethos for coping with infertility: a largely unconditional acceptance and appreciation for the various options available for people seeking "resolution." In the latter chapters of the book, I attempt to put my empirical data in sustained conversation with ethical arguments and explain the ways I was challenged to attend to individual experience and personal suffering and to integrate these observations into a more nuanced ethical account of ART. What emerges from this conversation between ethics and experience is an argument shaped by my initial concerns about social justice and the work / family problem but also extending beyond these motivating issues.

The book closes with constructive proposals that call for ethicists to pay closer attention to the experiences of people facing infertility and conversely for organizations such as RESOLVE to be more open to ethical perspectives that raise questions about social context and the pressures bearing on individual choice. RESOLVE avoids ethical issues in the use of ART and fails to raise awareness of structural and cultural problems, including work and family conflicts and consumerism. RESOLVE, like American society generally, is too easily persuaded by the rhetoric of individual choice, which diminishes the capacity for critical reflection. At the same time, by not paying attention to individual experience, ethicists miss the fact that people facing infertility often undergo a transformative process—one that does not necessarily encourage greater awareness of and concern for the common good but one that ultimately challenges dominant American myths about choice, control, and even consumerism. For better or worse, ART seems to play a critical role in this process, serving almost as a rite of passage.

ART has been criticized on many grounds, including that these technologies serve as an inadequate remedy for social and economic structures that pressure women to delay childbearing and, more broadly, undermine progress toward societal gender justice. ART has also been criticized for its purportedly negative effects on the family and parental attitudes toward children. Attention to the experiences of people facing infertility and the decision to use ART, however, combined with a responsive ethical analysis, shows that these criticisms are incomplete, both assuming too much and missing some of the most pressing ethical problems posed by ART.

RESOLVE, as a midlevel institution, plays a significant role in supporting people who face infertility and in creating a space for an ongoing conversation about ART. Listening carefully to particular conversations reveals both the impoverished moral vocabulary available for challenging the structural problems and cultural values that affect the use of ART and the richness of individual experience in coping with and interpreting the meaning of insurmountable limits. My findings suggest that people facing infertility engage in a complex process of meaning making, including an almost religious reinterpretation of the limits posed by bodily existence in a culture that prizes autonomy and control. At the same time, the individualistic assumptions embedded in the institutional and cultural setting of ART prevent people from engaging in ethical reflection on issues of justice, including the larger social and economic causes of the issues with which they are struggling.

ONE

Questions in the Abstract
Assisted Reproductive Technologies as
Private Choice and Social Practice

Background

What Are Assisted Reproductive Technologies?

Assisted reproduction is not a new phenomenon, but the cluster of tech-nologies now commonly referred to as assisted reproductive technologies or, more recently, advanced reproductive technologies (ART) dates only to the late 1970s. Dr. Patrick Steptoe and Dr. Robert Edwards performed the first successful in vitro fertilization (IVF) of a human embryo that was sustained through a normal pregnancy and resulted in a live birth, that of Louise Brown in July 1978 in Great Britain. IVF was a breakthrough technology that cir-cumvented some types of female infertility, including blocked fallopian tubes, the physiological problem that prevented Louise Brown's mother, Lesley, from conceiving. Other types of lower-tech assisted reproduction, such as artificial insemination, had long been used successfully, but IVF was some-thing new. After another successful IVF was performed in the United States, researchers and doctors on both sides of the Atlantic rapidly developed and applied the procedure throughout the 1980s and 1990s.

ART encompasses not only the IVF procedure, where fertilization of egg and sperm takes place outside the body and the few-day-old embryo is im-planted in the woman's uterus, but also a few variations. To be precise, the U.S. Centers for Disease Control and Prevention defines ART as "all treat-ments or procedures that involve surgically removing eggs from a woman's ovaries and combining the eggs with sperm to help a woman become pregnant. The types of ART are in vitro fertilization, gamete intrafallopian transfer, and zygote intrafallopian transfer."[1] In the case of IVF, the egg is fertilized outside the body and the resulting zygote or embryo is placed directly into the wom-an's uterus through her cervix, usually on day 5 of the embryo's development.

IVF provides the ability to document that fertilization occurred and the opportunity to evaluate embryo quality. The vast majority of ART cycles use IVF. In gamete intrafallopian transfer (GIFT), the eggs and sperm are combined outside the body but placed together inside the fallopian tube, the natural site of fertilization, through small incisions in a woman's abdomen. GIFT differs from IVF in that fertilization takes place inside the body. In zygote intrafallopian transfer (ZIFT), the egg is fertilized outside the body and the resulting zygote is placed in the fallopian tube, rather than the uterus, through small incisions in a woman's abdomen.[2]

In all types of ART, fertilization takes place without sexual intercourse. A woman's ovaries are stimulated through a regimen of drugs that cause multiple eggs to mature at the same time, a process called superovulation. After the eggs are surgically retrieved, the woman's uterus is then prepared for pregnancy (technically, the implantation of an embryo in the uterine lining) through the administration of a progesterone supplement. If an adequate number of eggs cannot be retrieved or if a woman experiences the symptoms of hyperstimulation, the drugs may be discontinued and the ART cycle canceled.[3] However, in most cases, the cycle moves forward, and the retrieved eggs are combined with sperm and transferred back into the woman's body.

ART does not encompass such lower-tech methods of assisted reproduction as artificial insemination, intrauterine insemination, or the various hormonal drug therapies available to women to increase the likelihood of conception (for example, Clomid). ART also does not encompass the many medical treatments for health problems that can cause infertility (for example, surgery to treat endometriosis in a woman or to repair a varicocele in a man). ART is considered high tech because it involves sophisticated surgical and laboratory procedures, including the surgical retrieval of eggs from the woman's ovaries, which is performed under intravenous sedation; the grading and manipulation of eggs and sperm in the laboratory; and the transferring of embryos or gametes back to the woman's body, typically an outpatient procedure performed without anesthesia.

Although most ART cycles use fresh, nondonor eggs or embryos, other applications of ART also exist. For example, many couples use cryopreservation after an IVF cycle to freeze or save extra embryos for later attempts to become pregnant. Couples increasingly combine IVF with the use of an egg donor or embryo donor. In these cases, the donor undergoes the egg retrieval procedure and the intended mother undergoes the transfer procedure. A smaller number of people combine IVF with a gestational surrogate. In this case, the intended mother may undergo the egg retrieval procedure or may use a donor, and the surrogate undergoes the transfer procedure.

In addition, several micromanipulation techniques increase the chances of a successful fertilization. For example, a refinement of IVF involves intra-cytoplasmic sperm injection (ICSI), in which a single sperm is physically injected into an egg to cause fertilization. ICSI is beneficial when there is male-factor infertility such as low sperm count or poor sperm quality. It has also been used to increase fertilization rates in older women and in women whose eggs have thick outer walls.[4]

An even newer procedure, cytoplasmic transfer, seeks to revitalize old eggs by combining the nucleus of an older woman's egg (that is, the egg of the woman trying to become pregnant) with the cytoplasm of a younger woman's egg (that is, the donor). The resulting embryo is thought to be healthier and more likely to implant in the uterus, but it may also contain genetic material from both eggs because the mitochondria in the younger egg's cytoplasm contain genetic material. Although cytoplasmic transfer has resulted in the birth of a few live babies, the procedure remains highly experimental and is not yet widely available.[5] Indeed, in 2001 the U.S. Food and Drug Administration (FDA) intervened and required clinicians at St. Barnabas Hospital in Livingston, New Jersey, one of the first U.S. clinics to attempt cytoplasmic transfer, to submit an Investigational New Drug application before proceeding with cytoplasmic transfer. The FDA's intervention effectively halted the procedure, as most practitioners around the country did not want to submit to the application process.[6]

Despite their complexity, all of the techniques that fall under the rubric of ART are still accurately thought of as variations, refinements, or combinations of the original IVF technology with other technologies. ART has opened up a whole new world of treatment possibilities for people experiencing infertility.

ART in the United States Today

According to the national registry, about forty-one U.S. clinics performed ART in 1986.[7] Since then, the number of clinics has increased significantly. According to the "2002 Assisted Reproductive Technology Success Rates: National Summary and Fertility Clinic Report" (the ART Report, a national summary of success rates published each year by the Centers for Disease Control and Prevention), the United States had 428 ART clinics in 2002, with 391 of them submitting data.[8] Most clinics are located in or near major cities— New York and metro Los Angeles each has more than ten clinics.[9] The Atlanta area, where I did my research, also has several prominent fertility clinics.

Approximately 6.2 million American women, or about 10 percent of those in their childbearing years, experience infertility, which is commonly defined as the inability to conceive after one year of unprotected intercourse.[10] According to statistics gathered by the National Survey of Family Growth, the absolute number of women experiencing fertility problems increased from 5.5 million in 1988 to 6.7 million in 1995, in part because of the aging baby boom generation.[11] During this same period, the absolute number of women who had ever sought medical help for fertility problems grew by 30 percent, from 2.1 million to 2.7 million.[12] However, not all women who experience fertility problems seek medical help. According to the statistics gathered in 1995, 42 percent of women with fertility problems had used infertility services.[13] The most common services reported were advice (60 percent), diagnostic tests (50 percent), medical help to prevent miscarriage (44 percent), and ovulation drugs (35 percent). Fewer than 2 percent of women seeking infertility services used ART.[14]

In the United States, the members of this select group tend to be older, to be married, to have college educations, to have high incomes, and to be white. Two demographers recently performed a multivariate analysis with data from the National Survey of Family Growth. By controlling for factors such as education and income, they pinpointed which characteristics were most clearly associated with using infertility services. The researchers found that race and age, by themselves, are less clearly associated with using infertility services than are having been "married, having higher levels of income and education, and having been covered by private health insurance in the last twelve months."[15] Elizabeth Hervey Stephen and Anjani Chandra further explain that they "hypothesize that race and ethnicity, to the extent that they serve as a proxy for socioeconomic status, may now distinguish those who can afford 'higher end' or specialized services."[16] Thus, this analysis supports the interpretation that socioeconomic status is a very important predictor of ART use and a more definitive predictor of ART use than race or age alone. Stephen and Chandra also note that marital status, "which is strongly correlated with having private insurance and higher income, is likely a proxy for an entire set of behaviors that are associated with infertility service-seeking."[17]

Most health insurance plans do not cover treatments for infertility, so the cost of ART is borne largely out of pocket. According to the American Society of Reproductive Medicine, the average cost of a single cycle of IVF in the United States is about $12,000.[18] However, additional costs are associated with an IVF pregnancy. According to one 1994 study, "On average, the cost incurred per successful delivery with in vitro fertilization increases from $66,667 for the first cycle of IVF to $114,286 by the sixth cycle. The cost increases because with each cycle in which fertilization fails, the probability that a subsequent effort will be successful declines."[19] The cost is lower for couples with a better chance of success, but for older couples with more difficult infertility problems (that is, the woman is older than forty and male-factor infertility also exists), the cost of a successful delivery ranges from $160,000 for the first cycle to $800,000 by the sixth. In the past few years, many clinics have instituted "shared-risk" or refund programs to patients without health insurance. In these programs, patients pay a higher fee up front to receive a fixed number of ART cycles (for example, three) but receive a substantial refund if no pregnancy or delivery occurs.[20]

Success rates for ART depend on a number of variables, including most significantly the age of the woman undergoing treatment if she is using her own eggs. Since the passage of the 1992 Fertility Clinic Success Rate and Certification Act, U.S. fertility clinics are required to report their success rates to the Centers for Disease Control and Prevention. The annual ART Reports have consistently shown that rates of pregnancy and live births are relatively high for women in their twenties but decline for women in their early thirties and drop more sharply from the mid-thirties onward. For example, in 1999, the percentage of ART cycles (using fresh embryos from nondonor eggs) resulting in live births was 32.2 percent for women under thirty-five, 26.2 percent for women ages thirty-five to thirty-seven, 18.5 percent for women thirty-eight to forty, and 9.7 percent for women forty-one or forty-two.[21] The 2002 ART Report, which examines trends in ART use from 1996 to 2002, notes that success rates improved for all age groups. Even so, some 65 percent of ART cycles using fresh nondonor eggs in 2002 did not result in a pregnancy. Just shy of 1 percent resulted in ectopic pregnancies, which are not viable, while 19.9 percent resulted in single-fetus pregnancies, 12.4 percent resulted in multiple-fetus pregnancies, and 2 percent ended in miscarriage.[22] Fewer than 83 percent of the viable pregnancies resulted in live births.[23]

In addition to age, other factors affecting success rates include whether the embryos were created from nondonor or donor eggs and whether the embryos are fresh or frozen. The success rates with fresh embryos are uniformly higher than with frozen, and the success rate using fresh embryos created from donor eggs is the highest of all types of ART cycles. (Donor eggs are typically taken from women in their twenties and thirties.) The average rate of live births per transfer using fresh embryos created from donor eggs is about 50 percent. The age of the woman receiving the donated egg does not materially affect success, so this statistic includes women of all ages (including those older than forty-two).[24] By contrast, when ART cycles use a woman's own eggs, the rate of live births declines precipitously with age: for example, to 4.0 percent at age forty-four and 1.2 percent at age forty-six.[25]

Finally, the trend of increased fertility problems appears to be associated with the factor of delayed childbearing. Women aged between thirty-five and forty-four make up 36 percent of the general population of women but 43 percent of the women reporting fertility problems. The difference is even more pronounced among nulliparous women (those who have never had a child): nulliparous women aged thirty-five to forty-four comprise 16 percent of the general population of women but 36 percent of the women reporting fertility problems.[26] Women clearly are waiting longer to have their first children. According to one source, the rate of first births for women in their thirties and forties has quadrupled since 1970.[27]

Although ART does not threaten to replace unassisted reproduction any time soon, it is growing in popularity among a certain group of Americans, some of whom attempt multiple cycles of IVF in their quests to overcome infertility. Between 1996 and 2002, for example, the total number of ART cycles performed grew from 64,681 to 115,392—an increase of 78 percent.[28] ART is also responsible for the lives of many children: the number of babies born through ART increased a dramatic 120 percent during those same years, from 20,840 in 1996 to 45,751 in 2002.[29] Finally, the increasing use of ART bears partial responsibility for the huge success of the infertility industry, which now grosses $4 billion per year.[30]

Ethical Questions

Since its introduction in the United States in the early 1980s, ART has generated and continues to generate diverse moral questions and answers. Within the fields of philosophical and religious ethics, feminist ethics, and biomedical ethics broadly defined, the responses have run the gamut from enthusiastic embrace to intense objection. The complex factors and distinct normative values on which these responses are based do not represent fixed or immovable points of reference so much as evolving perspectives in an ongoing scholarly conversation. I locate my particular perspective within this conversation as a means of raising what I consider to be relevant ethical questions about ART and the infertility industry.

I draw my point of view from theoretical perspectives within biomedical ethics, feminist ethics, and philosophical and religious ethics. My deeper roots, however, lie in feminist ethics and Christian ethics—in particular, in their overlapping areas of interest. To illustrate the areas of concern shared by feminist ethics and Christian ethics, I engage the work of Lisa Cahill, a feminist Christian (or Christian feminist). Cahill simultaneously attends to the social context of ART, including the cultural value of autonomy that supports its use, and ART's impact on the well-being of women, children, marriages, families, and most broadly the common good. I share with Cahill a willingness to explore the "final ends" of ART—what these technologies are for, whom they serve, and to what good or ill effects. Like Cahill, I draw from feminism in asking what best serves women's interests and from a religiously informed perspective in asking what best promotes human flourishing. What distinguishes my work is its methodological commitment to attend to the lived experience of infertility and to incorporate that experience into an ethical analysis.

Attending to the lived experience of infertility does not mean simply reporting data about ART and its users in the early-twenty-first-century United States. I do not think any researcher can report neutrally on a social phenomenon without letting his or her normative values frame the project.[31] In my investigation of ART, I have asked questions that assume there are better and worse choices, not simply greater or fewer numbers of choices. This chapter seeks to describe more fully my values and commitments and thus to identify the lens through which I interpret the social world of people using ART.

What Is the Purpose of ART?

To me, the most striking problem raised by ART is that, simply put, we do not seem to know what it is for. Like most technological advances, ART seems "good" because it solves a problem: the inability to conceive a child of one's own. However, what ART does and what this means is far more ambiguous than is typically acknowledged.

The ambiguity of assisted reproduction in many ways epitomizes a larger confusion about the general goals of medicine: Should physicians, as members of a time-honored profession with traditionally coherent moral commitments, seek to heal illness and relieve suffering, or are physicians now better understood as well-trained technicians available for hire in a morally pluralistic world, expected to promote the autonomous wishes of their consumer-patients without much comment? This question has been the subject of discussion within the medical ethics community for well over a decade because it epitomizes the challenge of moral pluralism in the context of contemporary medicine.[32] Different people have different views about the legitimacy of using growth hormones on short but otherwise healthy children, for example, just as they have different ideas about the legitimacy of breast implants or the appropriateness of hastening the death of someone facing a terminal illness.

Assisted reproduction is just one of many areas where what the patient desires may not necessarily fit neatly into the domain of traditional medicine. When does ART treat an illness, and when does it enable the expression of an individual patient's autonomous desires to procreate according to his or her personal values (for example, a single man who hires a surrogate mom or an older couple who hires an Ivy League egg donor)?[33] When, if ever, should a physician challenge what a patient wants, even if that goal has very little chance of being realized, as long as the patient has been informed of the risks and willingly consents to them? These questions have no easy answers in a context where the principle of autonomy has become the paramount arbiter of moral conflicts and where what serves the "patient's good" is generally assumed to be something that only the patient can authentically decide for him- or herself.

Despite the strong pull of autonomy as a dominant cultural value and a dominant concept in bioethics, reasons to challenge its preeminence still exist. Debate continues about the limits of patient autonomy and the proper ends of medicine, and debate about the limits of patient autonomy in the area of reproduction—specifically, women's reproductive freedom—is particularly intense. Many observers have criticized the trend of expecting physicians to be merely technicians for hire, with no independent moral compass. For physicians to acquiesce to patient demands can seem like abdicating responsibility for the patient's good, a deeper commitment that many people believe provides the moral core of the medical profession. At the same time, other critics plausibly assert that the ability to choose the timing and manner through which one procreates (like the ability to choose the timing and manner of one's own death) lies at the very heart of personal liberty and therefore trumps the seemingly antiquated virtues of medical paternalism.

In the midst of this ongoing debate enter the impressive technological advancements of reproductive medicine. Every year brings new developments and improved success rates. And each advancement, whatever its intended purpose or the particular medical problem it was designed to overcome, opens the door to numerous applications and consequences, some anticipated, others not. For example, the next "breakthrough" technology on the horizon of assisted reproduction, egg freezing (the physical removal and cryopreservation of human oocytes or eggs), "also might allow women to delay their reproductive choices, or enable some of them to preserve their ovarian tissue before undergoing treatments such as cancer chemotherapy, that could threaten their reproductive health. . . . In the future, as the difficulties of freezing and thawing eggs are overcome, it is probable that egg freezing will slowly join the mainstream of assisted reproductive technologies—most likely in the area of egg donation. And when this technology is perfected, women and their families and physicians will have another valuable option for treating infertility."[34] This discussion exemplifies the kind of ambiguity that cries out for further clarification. The article's author writes that egg freezing could accomplish a variety of goals but does not explicitly justify any of them: it preserves fertility when a woman must undergo a fertility-jeopardizing medical treatment; it allows women to delay childbearing by saving healthy oocytes for later use; it allows fertility clinics to store donated eggs; and it "treats" infertility, although how egg freezing is a treatment for existing (not future) infertility is especially unclear.

The author uses the more established legitimacy of medical treatment to lend legitimacy to all the potential uses of egg freezing, thereby helping to bring this new technology into the mainstream. No one would deny the obvious medical benefit of allowing a woman to receive life-saving chemotherapy and preserve her fertility through egg freezing. Yet there is no attempt to argue for the legitimacy of the other uses of egg freezing, including the ability to "delay reproductive choices," other than to phrase it in terms of creating more options and greater choice.[35]

Is ART fundamentally about the treatment of an illness, or is it fundamentally about serving other goals, such as the need or desire to delay childbearing? Is it both? Why should it matter whether society comes to any kind of consensus about the purpose of egg freezing or any other use of ART? My discussion of the hypothetical career pill (ostensibly a chemical version of egg freezing) should clearly demonstrate that I consider ART's boundaries rather amorphous. This lack of definition is problematic ethically because more is at stake in the use of ART than the expression of individual consumer preferences. I view the use of ART not simply as a private choice affecting only the individual who uses it but as a social practice with broader consequences—for women generally, for children and families, and for future generations. The use of ART is also a social practice in the sense that it grows out of a specific set of social and historical circumstances that deserve further scrutiny.

That many women desire "to delay their reproductive choices" and that this desire is perceived to grow out of a legitimate set of circumstances creates the implicit link between ART as "treatment" and ART as "elective procedure." There may be a compelling argument why the elective use of egg freezing to preserve future reproductive options in an otherwise healthy woman is every bit as legitimate as the use of ART to treat existing infertility, but the author of this article does not make the case. In fact, the literature promoting ART rarely makes the case. However, the social conditions favoring delayed childbearing should not be equated with the physical illnesses or disabilities that cause infertility. To use the language of philosopher Judith Shklar, the latter might be considered a misfortune, while the former might be better thought of as an injustice.[36] If we fail to recognize the constructed nature of the conditions favoring delayed childbearing, we lose any inclination to question whether those conditions are just. Indeed, the perception that individuals' choices—especially in the area of reproduction—are disconnected from a larger social context and from concerns about justice encourages a certain moral complacency with regard to ART's many potential uses. Reproductive choices are thought to represent only individuals' best interests and most private desires.

How Does ART Relate to Delayed Childbearing?

Two significant and commonly discussed changes in work have dramatically affected American society: more women have paid employment than ever before, and many Americans, both men and women, feel they are overworked. Both of these statements require elaboration and qualification.

Much has been made of the enormous influx of women into the workforce over the last few decades of the twentieth century. Observers often point out that women of color have always worked outside the home in greater proportion than white women and that these working women of color have managed to combine work and family responsibilities out of necessity. Indeed, only recently have maternal employment rates for different racial ethnic groups begun to converge. Most mothers, both white and nonwhite, work outside the home: maternal employment has tripled over the past thirty years, increasing steadily for all racial ethnic groups.[37] But nonwhite working mothers continue to work longer hours and for less money than their white counterparts.[38]

Second, people are working harder than ever. Juliet Schor's *The Overworked American* (1992) went a long way toward raising awareness about the amount of time Americans devote to work. Using statistics from the late 1960s to the late 1980s, she finds that the average employed person now works an extra month (163 hours) per year. She also finds a gender gap in the work increase: men are doing 98 more hours per year and women are doing a staggering 305 more hours per year.[39] Studies also show that even mothers who work outside the home remain the primary caretakers of children and the household.[40]

Like the influx of women into paid employment, the observation that Americans are overworked needs to be qualified. Sociologists Jerry Jacobs and Kathleen Gerson argue that overwork exists primarily for the professional and middle classes but that significant underwork or unemployment exists for other groups.[41] Their findings corroborate Ellen Goodman's observation that "we seem to be evolving into two classes, the underemployed and the overemployed, those who are desperate for work and those who are desperate for time."[42]

Alongside problems with the structure of work are problems with the structure of families. The increase in maternal employment (or at least the increase in white middle-class maternal employment) and the phenomenon of over-work (or at least the overworked middle and professional classes) have together spawned a great deal of theorizing about the structuring effects of gender and the gendered division of labor. Our society apparently has been slow to adjust to the reality of working mothers. Little has changed with regard to our expectations of mothers' duties in the home or with regard to wage earners' productivity in a competitive economy.[43] Briefly put, "Two-earner families are trying to do something in a world that's designed for one-earner families."[44]

Although expectations about families and women's duties to family may not have changed much in recent decades, noticeable changes in childbearing practices have occurred. Childbearing takes place later than in previous decades, and birthrates have declined.[45] In the professional class, many women delay childbearing until their careers are well established.[46] The significance of these trends with regard to the increased use of ART is by no means self-evident. The best data available suggest that income, education, and marital status are among the characteristics most strongly associated with the use of ART. If any relationship exists between the increased use of ART and conditions favoring delayed childbearing, what may be the most plausible interpretation is that ART is functioning not to alleviate the strain between work and family experienced by millions of American families of different social classes but rather to expand reproductive options for a select, privileged group of women. Perhaps for this group, ART enables conception later in life, after professional goals have been attained.

However, it is always important to remember that the causes of infertility are varied and complex and cannot be attributed solely to delayed childbearing. In fact, some of the most significant risk factors for infertility include poor health care and untreated sexually transmitted diseases. Any feminist—or any person—concerned with the well-being of women would have to ask whether ART helps women whose infertility is caused by these problems.

Does ART Promote Women's Well-Being?

To date, the largest body of literature addressing ART has come from feminist scholars who recognized early on that assisted reproduction potentially affects women's health and well-being. As their work clearly illustrates, ART also intersects with women's roles as mothers, the institution of the family, the relationship of sexual difference to sexual equality, and the roles technology and consumerism can play in liberating and/or exploiting women. Precisely how ART intersects with these issues is open to different interpretations, and at no time were the responses within feminism more polarized than in the 1980s, when ART was first being used in the United States.[47]

Although no single representative feminist position on ART exists, the Feminist International Network of Resistance to Reproductive and Genetic Engineering (FINRRAGE) was very influential in setting the agenda for the initial feminist discussion. Scholars associated with FINRRAGE vocally opposed ART, believing these technologies to be highly exploitative of women as a group.[48] In her helpful historical overview, Anne Donchin describes the FINRRAGE position, sometimes referred to as "radical noninterventionist":[49] "The FINRRAGE program calls for suppressing the development and application of fertility technologies despite claims of many women that they provide the only means available to them to fulfill their procreative desires. The dissemination of these technologies, they insist, only reinforces women's oppression, giving scientific and therapeutic support to the patriarchal presumption that reproduction is a woman's prime commodity."[50] The skepticism that FINRRAGE feminists brought to reproductive technologies grew out of their deep suspicion of the medical establishment and its long history of disempowering women and women's experience of reproduction. FINRRAGE feminists pointed out the experimental nature of ART and contended that women were serving as experimental subjects—with significant health risks—in the guise of therapy. Moreover, given the pressures on women in a sexist society to undertake motherhood, members of FINRRAGE believed that women who used ART were not "genuinely" choosing to do so. Although these feminists conceded that individual women might benefit from assisted reproduction, they strenuously maintained that ART should be disavowed for the good of the collective—that is, for "women as a social group."[51]

On the other side of the early feminist debate were scholars who enthusiastically embraced ART and its many possibilities. The godmother of this "radical interventionist" position was, most famously, Shulamith Firestone, who invoked the liberating potential of disembodied human reproduction several years before the advent of ART.[52] Real equality with men, she argued, could be achieved only by defeating biological destiny, and artificial reproduction (even extracorporeal gestation) could be a legitimate tool for accomplishing this goal. These views, even though they predated the first successful use of IVF, influenced the development of more optimistic interpretations of ART. Feminists who understand gender and reproduction to be socially constructed saw in ART the opportunity to reconstruct reproduction in entirely new ways and to encourage new forms of social organization that would benefit women. For these feminists, ART created "new possibilities in the relationship between women and their bodies, new ways of conceptualizing the family, and new ways of thinking about the social contribution of reproductive services."[53] Accordingly, from this perspective, ART served rather than undermined the collective good by constituting a tool for women's liberation.

Other feminists, also fairly classified as radical interventionists, supported the use of ART out of a more classically liberal position, advocating individuals' rights to reproductive freedom and self-determination. Access to ART expands the range of decisions women can make about reproduction, these liberal feminists argued, increasing flexibility and choice. They also argued that ART enables women "to enter into collaborative contracts, to sell gametes or gestational services, or to bear children outside the confines of heterosexual marriage,"[54] thus increasing women's control over the fruits of their reproductive labor and power to enact their own diverse understandings of family and parenthood.

Finally, another group of voices embracing ART from the beginning includes advocates for the involuntarily infertile. Although they would not necessarily identify themselves as liberal feminists, advocates for the infertile similarly support ART for the benefits these technologies can provide to individual women. Supporters of this position are unconvinced that women's collective interests are served by suppressing the development and use of ART, believing it unfair to sacrifice the present interests of infertile women for future, dubious social goals.[55] Unlike adherents of the various feminist positions, advocates for the infertile are often labeled "pronatalist" rather than "feminist" because they tend to assume that the desire to procreate is natural, spontaneous, and not necessarily a sign of women's oppression. And in striking contrast to the FINRRAGE feminists, advocates for the infertile do not perceive women who use ART as passive victims of technology or the medical establishment. By FINRRAGE standards, advocates for the infertile are unconcerned with problems of false consciousness and instead view these women as exercising considerable self-determination in deciding to use ART and in striving to achieve their goals.

Some of the initial feminist responses to ART tended to oversimplify the issues. For example, *either* motherhood is the main source of women's oppression, and a technology that encourages "pronatalism" thus can only oppress women further, *or* motherhood is entirely natural and good, and a technology that assists in achieving legitimate procreative desires thus can only be a blessing. Many of the stronger anti- and pronatalist perspectives (as well as anti- and protechnology perspectives) still find expression in contemporary debates about ART, but some important developments and changes have also occurred, as has a general move toward greater complexity. A generation of feminist theorizing has challenged some of the early dichotomies between nature and culture, for example, and between feminist positions that prioritize only the collective or individual benefits/harms of using ART.

In her discussion of more recent feminist responses to ART, Donchin attributes these developments to three major themes in feminist theory that emerged in the 1990s: a reclamation of women's agency, a revaluation of mothering, and a more sophisticated appraisal of power relations.[56] She calls the FINRRAGE position "feminist fundamentalism" because it assumes that the general experience of a common oppression among women qualifies FINRRAGE to judge and even dictate the conduct of individual women. She also criticizes the FINRRAGE position because it denies the possibility of individual agency (that is, it claims that women choose ART out of irresistible pronatalist societal forces), denigrates the value of mothering (that is, it claims that mothering is closely connected to if not synonymous with the main sources of women's oppression in a patriarchal society), and assumes a simplistic picture of power relations (that is, it claims that women's reproductive experience rests largely in the hands of male doctors and/or husbands).

Donchin is equally critical of the other extreme, those who would give their unqualified support to individual decisions to use ART, especially advocates for the infertile who assume that an "individual woman's actions can be assessed in isolation from their social context," an assumption she finds politically naive.[57] In between feminist fundamentalism and pro-ART individualism, Donchin proposes a third alternative, "women who claim their desires as their own and, without disavowing the constraints of biology and social norms, still exercise self-determination."[58] According to this view, individual agency is not negated by social forces, motherhood is not the bane of women's existence, and users of ART should not be assumed to be victims operating out of false consciousness.

Most contemporary feminists occupy the middle ground described by Donchin, and it is a complex terrain.[59] Many contemporary feminists continue to criticize ART for a variety of reasons. Many support it with qualification. The nature/culture or embodiment/rationality debate seems to stand at the heart of some of these intrafeminist differences. Technology complicates the debate because, as a product of rationality, it can both threaten the "natural," such as the connections of biological-gestational-social parenthood, and mitigate natural inequalities, such as the fact that men are fertile for many more years than women. The question remains: Who wields the power of this technology, and to what end(s)?

Feminists, as feminists, share a concern for women's well-being, but considerable diversity of opinion exists about how to define women's well-being and about what promotes it. Historically, feminists have constructed some major philosophical frameworks for approaching these questions, but feminism has become more complex and nuanced over the past decade. The categories of liberal, radical, socialist, Marxist, postmodern, and other kinds of feminism, while still relevant, may be less decisive than was once the case. Martha Nussbaum, for example, is a liberal feminist philosopher who rejects elevating the collective good of any group (including the good of women as a group, families, communities, or nations) above the individual well-being and agency of group members. Yet she also retrieves from the liberal tradition the argument that individual freedom can be served only by tending to the social structures that make its expression possible. She simultaneously embraces "liberal individualism," which she defines as maximizing individual freedom and respect for individual worth, and a more typically "communitarian" concern for the common good.[60]

What divides contemporary feminists is not that some care about social goods and others do not but rather which social goods to support and how best to support them. Two distinct areas of disagreement arise in arguments about whether ART serves or undermines feminist social agendas: what these agendas or goals should be, and how this particular technology affects them. According to Maura Ryan, the social good of ART is ambiguous, especially with regard to whether it transforms human reproduction for the benefit of women: "The question of whether artificial reproduction can serve the social transformation of reproduction and reproductive choice is extremely complex. The fact that the advent of reproductive technology has proved to be a crisis for feminism—of social vision, of loyalty and ideological solidarity, of meaning and definition—is a testament to the importance of what is at stake."[61] One possible feminist response is that ART promotes the goal of redefining women's relationship to their bodies, which in turn can also promote the goal of sexual equality between men and women. ART makes human reproduction more of a volitional undertaking, giving women greater options, more control, and more time to combine career and motherhood.

As Ryan notes,

The more control women have over the manner and timing of reproduction, the more it is a personal accomplishment, an event which is undertaken and not simply suffered, and an intentional celebration of the immense creative and transformative power that is physical generativity. . . .

The radical version of this argument, that technology ought to be embraced as a means of freeing women from reproducing biologically altogether, has not found many supporters. But the availability of techniques in non-coital reproduction is a positive development if they allow women to overcome the biological clock, for example, to have both a career and a fulfilling parental experience.[62]

This relatively positive appraisal assumes that women, rather than the medical establishment or a patriarchal, pronatalist society, generally wield the power of ART. This view also assumes that ART can indeed overcome the biological clock and that doing so is desirable. Ryan's conclusions do not ultimately embrace this view, however. She argues instead that the only legitimate warrant for ART is as a health care claim, "as a medical treatment which addresses the personal anguish accompanying infertility," not an elective procedure to extend individual "procreative liberty" or to serve any particular feminist social goal.[63]

An alternative feminist response that Ryan does not develop in her argument holds that ART may indeed overcome the biological clock but that doing so in this manner is not necessarily a good thing. Such a view does not endorse a regressive "biology is destiny" naturalism but rather questions whether women wield the power of ART. This position takes a more negative view of how ART functions, arguing that it counters the feminist goals of sexual equality, justice, and adequate support of childbearing. For example, Laura Woliver argues that ART has become a technological means of allowing women to conform "equally" with men to modern capitalist timetables in education and employment.[64] According to this view, both women and men are now free to conform to structures that do not necessarily serve their own interests, benefit the interests of families, or contribute to the flourishing of the human community generally.[65]

Another major problem with ART is how it affects U.S. racial inequalities. In *Killing the Black Body: Race, Reproduction, and the Meaning of Liberty* (1997), Dorothy Roberts suggests that technological solutions can sometimes obscure social problems by leaving them unaddressed or passing them on to others: "Although the 'biological clock' metaphor is grossly exaggerated, one reason for infertility among white, educated, high-income women is their postponement of childbearing in order to pursue a career. The cause of these women's infertility is not biological; rather, it is a workplace that makes it virtually impossible for women to combine employment and child-rearing. These women can avoid this social problem by seeking expensive fertility treatment after achieving some status in the office."[66] As Roberts summarizes her argument, women "can afford to bypass the structural unfairness to mothers through technological intervention. Similarly, many affluent white women gained entry to the male-dominated workplace by assigning female domestic tasks to low-paid dark-skinned nannies."[67] Roberts expresses concern that expensive technological interventions may take the place of wider social reforms that could help resolve the conflicts between family and work for all women. Rather than serving feminist social goals, she believes, ART undermines efforts to restructure the workplace and the family so that participation of women and men of all races in both spheres could become more equitable.

The thesis that ART might provide a technological fix for structural injustices and that only some women have the opportunity to exploit the benefits of this fix is compelling because it offers a multidimensional interpretation of some of the ethical problems raised by ART.[68] This idea recognizes not only that ART expands individual freedom of choice, which may represent a real benefit for many women, but also that this expanded freedom of choice exacerbates many existing inequalities, including inequalities of class and race. In addition, this perspective suggests that technology constitutes a less than optimal solution for underlying social problems by diminishing the likelihood that lasting, transformative change will occur. It also places the burden of fixing a social problem on women's bodies.

The feminist critique of ART as a technological fix for social or structural problems may overemphasize a causal connection between the various factors contributing to the cultural trend of delayed childbearing and the increasing use of ART. The connection between delayed childbearing and increased fertility problems, while demonstrably accurate, does not logically require any one explanation for why women delay childbearing or choose to use ART rather than pursue some other alternative. Other causes of infertility must not be neglected, and the reasons why women might be drawn to ART in increasing numbers must not be oversimplified. Ignoring the complexity of these phenomena risks endorsing an overly narrow or reductive interpretation of ART, the women who use it, and the forces that make it attractive.

Does ART Expand Human Freedom?

In general, assisted reproduction is gaining wider acceptance in American society. Infertility is a booming industry in the United States, and the practices of IVF and the less high-tech artificial insemination are well established in many parts of the country. In addition to an increased demand for services, increased openness about infertility and infertility treatments has also developed. Prospective parents can acquire donor sperm through Internet catalogs, advertisements for donor eggs run in college newspapers and national magazines, and women willing to serve as surrogate mothers can meet infertile couples through surrogacy Web sites. Even the adoption process has moved toward greater openness, with biological and adoptive parents often meeting each other and maintaining contact throughout the child's life. These cultural changes, including society's increased comfort level and acceptance of a variety of procreative "choices," likely result (at least in part) from hard-won reproductive freedoms in other areas, including contraception and abortion rights. These protected freedoms are the fruit of major legal decisions as well as powerful philosophical arguments for procreative liberty.

A major, though underexplored, question in the literature on reproductive technologies is whether this increased freedom of choice equates with human flourishing. Are these concepts really synonymous? Moreover, what assumptions about the meaning of freedom and the meaning of human flourishing underlie our increased acceptance of reproductive technologies?

One definition of human freedom, which relies heavily on the assumptions of liberal individualism, comes from the work of John Robertson, a philosopher and legal scholar who has written widely on the subject of reproductive technologies. In his *Children of Choice: Freedom and the New Reproductive Technologies* (1994), Robertson examines different types of assisted reproduction (including artificial insemination, IVF, and surrogacy) as well as the issues of contraception, abortion, and nonreproductive uses of reproductive capacities (for example, research on embryos). He clearly advocates a standard presumption in favor of procreative liberty: unless there is a clear indication of tangible harm, people should be free to procreate when and how they please.

Robertson's strategy is to extend the more well-established right to avoid unwanted procreation to an analogous right to procreate when procreation is desired. This right to procreate, he then argues, should include the freedom to use technological assistance when it is needed to achieve the desired goal. Robertson reviews the legal protections of the right to avoid procreation, including the U.S. Supreme Court's 1972 *Eisenstadt v. Baird* decision, which claimed a constitutionally protected freedom to use contraception,[69] as well as the relevant Supreme Court decisions on abortion. Drawing on language from the Supreme Court's decision in *Planned Parenthood v. Casey* (1992), Robertson articulates a broader philosophical justification of procreative liberty: Because procreation is so important, so fundamental to the human experience, "involving the most intimate and personal choices a person may make in a lifetime, choices central to personal dignity and autonomy,"[70] individuals should neither be forced to undertake it nor deprived of the opportunity to accomplish it. If procreation cannot be achieved through sexual intercourse, the right to procreate should include the freedom to use technological assistance or the assistance of a third party (although no positive obligation exists on the part of the state to provide such assistance). According to Robertson, "If bearing, begetting, or parenting children is protected as part of personal privacy or liberty, those experiences should be protected whether they are achieved coitally or noncoitally."[71]

After so defining procreative liberty, Robertson weighs the benefits of this liberty against possible competing interests. Although he claims procreative liberty is not absolute, he believes it deserves "presumptive priority" because in most cases the competing interests do not rise to the level of "tangible harm" to others.[72] Robertson recognizes that the use of some reproductive technologies can occasion ambivalence and doubt, both for individuals and for society as a whole, but he believes that protecting liberty itself is the most important value in a free society such as ours.

Not unlike legal scholar Ronald Dworkin, who uses a similar strategy with abortion and euthanasia in *Life's Dominion: An Argument about Abortion, Euthanasia, and Individual Freedom* (1993), Robertson "privatizes" the issue of reproductive technologies as a means of defending their use.[73] Robertson claims that human reproduction is a matter of great personal significance and importance for an individual's sense of dignity and meaning. But human reproduction, according to Robertson, is foremost a private experience, one that individuals invest with private and diverse meanings. The state should not interfere with this experience unless tangible harm to others will result. "Merely symbolic" concerns, including religious and moral objections to separating sex and reproduction, "should not override the use of these techniques for forming a family."[74] That some people's sensibilities might be offended is not enough to constitute actual harm.

Robertson identifies himself as using consequentialist reasoning to weigh benefits and harms in the exercise of procreative liberty. He rejects out of hand deontological arguments about a "right way" of reproducing, claiming them to be fundamentally illegitimate as public arguments. Because reasonable people will differ in a pluralistic society about the "right way" to reproduce, moral concerns about reproduction are more appropriately resolved by private consciences. Robertson thus presents a typical, if almost caricatured, liberal defense of the so-called value-neutral public sphere and the priority of freedom of conscience.

Robertson's vision of the person—or what it means to be human—is grounded in a very strong view of autonomy. What matters when we decide to procreate is what we voluntarily will. Robertson states that we should honor the "prime movers" in all reproductive arrangements—those persons who decided to create a child using whatever collaborative means they desire.[75] Robertson also believes that assisted reproductive arrangements should be contractual and binding, implying that preferences and needs can be known ahead of time and are not subject to change. He is confident that parties to the contract will be able to make "free choices" provided that informed consent exists. Even concerns about social justice, whatever those might be (for example, it is unfair that access to ART is severely limited by its cost), do not constitute compelling enough reasons to limit procreative liberty.

What emerges from *Children of Choice* is a view of autonomy as the primary ethical value governing the use of reproductive technologies and as the primary characteristic of human beings. Other values, such as social justice or shared symbolic meanings, receive little weight. "Tangible harm" is taken to be literal harm to already existing persons, not to children that would have no other way of being born or to the wider community whose views about parenthood and the dignity of children might alter profoundly over time.

A striking contrast to Robertson's view of human freedom appears in the works of Cahill and Oliver O'Donovan, both of whom are better described as religious ethicists. Religious ethics has an enormous range, and O'Donovan and Cahill are only two voices within one religious tradition, Christianity. Still, they offer views of human freedom and human flourishing that provide an alternative to Robertson's singular emphasis on autonomy. They also suggest the diverse and complex ways that any religious tradition can be interpreted. For better or worse, the Christian perspective on assisted reproduction is often monolithically reduced to the Catholic Church's prohibition against separating procreation from the sex act in marriage.[76] This unequivocal prohibition is not, however, the final word on assisted reproduction from a Christian perspective—in either the Protestant or Catholic traditions.

For example, in his influential text, *Begotten or Made?* (1984), O'Donovan articulates what he believes to be at stake ethically in the use of assisted reproduction by focusing not on the autonomy of the adults who wish to procreate but on the relationship of parent and child.[77] All of O'Donovan's arguments are based on his interpretation of the Christian tradition as a person of faith (he is Protestant) and seem to be addressed to an audience that shares his point of view. Not necessarily compelled to make his arguments more generally or publicly persuasive, he concludes his chapters with explicit directives about how a Christian should proceed in these matters.[78]

Despite O'Donovan's somewhat insular approach (that is, his perspective of speaking to a community of like-minded believers), his insights have a wider applicability and have had lasting influence. In brief, his interpretation of assisted reproduction hinges on drawing a distinction between *praxis* (begetting) and *poesis* (making). Simply put, he states that human beings beget other human beings, but only God "makes" or creates human beings. The significance of this distinction is that only by begetting do we respect the dignity of the begotten as a being of equal moral worth, as another "I" with a distinct personality and destiny.[79] Only by begetting do we treat the child as an end in itself rather than a means to our own ends. O'Donovan explicitly grounds this view in a faith in God: Because of the equality of humanity before God, all human beings are understood to be on an equal moral plane with each other.

The problem with *poesis*, he argues, is that it alienates the product from its maker. We can never be on equal moral ground with that which is the object of our art or craft because it is subject to our will. This alienation can alter the meaning of parenthood and attitudes toward children, promoting the idea that children serve as means to adult fulfillment and self-definition. Lost is the idea that children are gifts—more explicitly, gifts from God—for which we have special responsibility or stewardship. What is feared is that children might come to be seen as objects or commodities that unfortunately cannot be returned or exchanged if they disappoint parental expectations.

O'Donovan's analysis begs the question of what exactly constitutes "making" in the realm of assisted reproduction. We do not want to treat children as means to adult ends, but how does any kind of assisted reproduction promote that attitude? O'Donovan sees as problematic the use of a third-party donor (sperm or egg) and/or gestational surrogate, not necessarily the use of a medical technology that enables conception to occur, such as IVF by itself. He contends that when we separate biological (including genetic and/or gestational) parenthood from social parenthood, we move closer to "making" rather than begetting our children. When we break that connection with biology, we undermine our knowledge of what it means to be a parent. Being a parent, according to O'Donovan, is something more than whoever freely chooses to assume that role.

O'Donovan's preference for *praxis* over *poesis* as a way of understanding human reproduction is based on his belief that our knowledge possesses a "natural substrate." Like the papal encyclicals on assisted reproduction, O'Donovan's writings seek to articulate the value or the dignity of procreation as an embodied good. One lives in one's body and experiences bodily existence. The givenness of the body and the biological processes of reproduction are part of the created order. However, as human beings, we are always more than mere biology. O'Donovan ultimately draws the line in a different place than does the Vatican—he is open to certain forms of assisted reproduction where the Vatican is not—but he similarly tries to retain the idea that the bodily has moral significance. Unlike Robertson, who exclusively prioritizes the volitional, O'Donovan attempts to make room for that which is not chosen in life and for the good of embodied existence, believing these to be part of full human flourishing.

For O'Donovan, assisted reproduction's threat ultimately lies in the threat of a technological culture in which it becomes harder and harder to think in categories that are not artificial, that are not driven by means/ends instrumental calculation.[80] If everything is taken to be "made" or constructed, the category of "natural" becomes evacuated of meaning. Thus, O'Donovan maintains that we need to accord respect to nature—whether that be respect for the natural environment or respect for human reproduction—to avoid undermining the conditions that make life possible.

One final concern raised by O'Donovan pertains to the impact of assisted reproduction on future generations. Decisions to use assisted reproduction—with or without third-party donors, cryopreservation, or micromanipulation techniques—are never only about the current decision makers but always implicate the well-being of future persons. O'Donovan points to the injustice of taking risks on behalf of the health of future persons who have no way to hold accountable those responsible. Others make the case that the logic of these technologies leads to eugenics.[81] Just as parents have special responsibilities toward individual children, so too does society have special obligations to the human society of tomorrow, including the health of the human gene pool. These arguments rest on potentially more generalizable views of justice and reciprocity but also find roots in Judeo-Christian values about how human beings ought to treat each other and interact with the natural world.

Does ART Promote Human Flourishing?

Like O'Donovan, Cahill's interest in ART extends considerably beyond the subject of whether it promotes the individual autonomy of its adult users. Cahill's singularly incisive critique of ART (and of our times) is not that technology is "bad" and only "natural" procreation is good but that the way we consume infertility services, the way we choose ART without a broader societal conversation about the significance of what we are doing, and the way the infertility industry generally resists regulation are signs of our society's elevation of "choice" itself as a nearly absolute value. It is the elevation of individual autonomy without regard for the embodied and social dimensions of human experience. Cahill is particularly worried that a lack of critical discussion about the "final values or ends for which reproductive clients act" will leave room for the "still strong forces of patriarchy and market economics . . . to govern 'autonomous' reproductive choice."[82]

A feminist scholar working out of the tradition of Catholic social ethics, Cahill combines an interest in both the social context of ART and the moral significance of "private" decisions to use it. She specifies what she believes are the goods of marriage and parenthood and discusses how assisted reproduction, including the use of third-party donors, may affect them. Her book, *Sex, Gender, and Christian Ethics* (1996) seeks to construct an overarching Christian feminist sexual ethic that has sexual equality as one of its core values yet also retains the Catholic commitment to embodiment and sociality. She uses the case of ART to illustrate some of the key features of this ethic.

Cahill, like O'Donovan, places ART in the larger context of a vision for human flourishing, asking specifically whether certain uses of this technology promote such flourishing. For example, Cahill does not endorse egg donation simply because it gives infertile women and older women more options, nor does she approve of sex selection simply because it gives parents greater control over and thus greater satisfaction in the composition of their families. While there is nothing inherently wrong with expanding one's options, we must also ask whether creating a child through the use of a third-party donor or creating a child according to our preferred sex at the time of conception truly contributes to the flourishing of the child, the parents, and human society generally. These questions are legitimate and important but are obscured by the rhetoric of choice.

Of course, Cahill is well aware that not everyone is interested in her vision of human flourishing and the place of ART within it. She recognizes that the rhetoric of choice has to some extent evolved as a reaction against oppressive "visions of human flourishing." Indeed, she knows that many people are skeptical that any vision at all of human flourishing can be shared, so thoroughly have our normative foundations been shaken by postmodernism. But Cahill is unwilling to retire the concept of human flourishing. Mindful of the formidable challenges posed by postmodern thinking, Cahill nevertheless aims to develop a normative Christian feminist ethic of sex and reproduction. She believes she can describe this ethic in a way that is publicly accessible, that she can be forthright about the faith commitments that underpin this ethic without undermining its integrity or persuasiveness, and that her voice and all religious voices ought to have a role in shaping the common good. She believes that the facts of pluralism and diversity do not make it impossible to derive some universalizable norms that are based on shared human needs and that seek to achieve human flourishing.[83] She is not persuaded by the argument that power determines values and that values are no more than whatever the prevailing views of the day may be.

How does she arrive at this position? Cahill uses critical realism to develop her normative ethic of sex and reproduction. Specifically, she works out of the Aristotelian-Thomistic natural law tradition, using its inductive approach to build norms from empirical reality.[84] This is not to say that she takes the category of "natural" as a simple, self-evident given. Cahill looks at both bodily realities and the social constructions that people in different cultures give to those bodily realities, asking whether these constructions necessarily depend on the body. For example, the fact that females give birth does not justify sexual discrimination. She also asks whether existing human institutions (for example, marriage) contribute to human flourishing.

Cahill has a great deal at stake in reclaiming a view of bodily experience as a real phenomenon that cannot be wholly collapsed into or explained by social construction. She is committed to affirming the good of creation and the good of bodily experience. She is committed to upholding the basic relational nature and sociality of human beings. And she is committed to avoiding the common slippage into mind/body dualism, which she believes is the particular vice of the "ideology of choice." She defines the ideology of choice as a tendency, especially prevalent in American culture, to absolutize the value of autonomy while neglecting other legitimate values. Cahill's commitments, which she identifies explicitly as Catholic commitments, lead her to question attempts to subordinate the bodily aspects of parenthood to its intentional or volitional aspects.

Despite her clear ties with natural law ethics, Cahill criticizes the Catholic Church for basing its disapproval of reproductive technologies on an insistence on procreative unity in each and every sex act.[85] Parting company with the Vatican, Cahill does not condemn all forms of ART. She carefully delineates those forms that she thinks contribute to human flourishing and those that do not. She draws an important distinction, as the Vatican does not, between types of assisted reproduction that use the couple's own gametes (that is, sperm and eggs) and types of ART that use third-party egg and/or sperm donors. Cahill finds acceptable the use of a technology to assist a couple in having a child as long as a third-party donor is not introduced into the relationship.[86] "Laboratory conception" by itself does not violate the sexually expressed love relationship of a couple, according to Cahill.

In taking this position, Cahill tries to strike a reasonable balance between the bodily and other important aspects of human existence. The physical experiences of sex and parenthood do have normative meaning, but that meaning is not absolute. Cahill writes, "The physical or embodied aspects of marriage and parenthood are not as important morally as those which are psychospiritual and social, which is why sexual intercourse is not a morally necessary means of conception."[87] Cahill believes an absolute ban on assisted reproduction does not adequately honor the larger context of a relationship, which can encompass both the procreative and unitive aspects of marriage over time and in different ways.

Cahill draws the line at third-party donors because she believes that the connections among genetic, gestational, and social parenthood constitute an ideal worth retaining for those who are reasonably able to meet it. This ideal is not meant to exclude or punish, she claims. The ideal is compelling because holding these aspects of parenthood together is good for both the parents and for the child. It is good for the parents because it preserves symmetry in their relationship, among other reasons. It is good for the child because biological kinship is an important (if not all-important) aspect of personal identity. Cahill treats adoption separately from the issue of assisted reproduction with third-party donors, primarily because adoption does not involve intentionally severing the connection with the genetic or biological parent as part of the process of achieving conception.[88] Cahill summarizes her normative position by declaring the biological component of parenthood and of personhood "subsidiary" to social components, but it remains important. When the connections among genetic, gestational, and social parenthood are deliberately severed, the biological component receives too little weight. Producing children becomes a matter of willful intentions and is "disembodied."[89] Cahill sees that something important is lost when freedom of the will triumphs completely over the body, and the loss is more than sentimental, fundamentally altering how human life is valued.

I do not wholeheartedly accept the balance Cahill strikes between honoring the volitional and embodied aspects of parenthood, even while I appreciate her effort to hold these two together and reclaim the importance of "embodied autonomy." A troubling vulnerability in her argument is the inherently subjective appraisal involved in discerning when enough weight has been given to the bodily or the biological. This judgment seems impossible in the abstract, and it inevitably involves excluding some people who are unable—for whatever reason—to hold the genetic, gestational, and social aspects of parenthood together.

Nevertheless, if any merit whatsoever exists in Cahill's argument for universalizable norms based on shared human needs and aimed at achieving human flourishing, it would be important to check our society's evolving comfort level with manipulating human reproduction against the actual well-being of children who result from ART, their parents, and human society generally. Cahill attempts to articulate a substantive vision of human flourishing that is not thoroughly relative. We would do well to continue to debate the precise weight that ought to be given to biological ties.

Moreover, and perhaps more importantly, since we are free to disagree with the reasons she gives for her position on third-party donors, Cahill's most relevant point may be the more general one that when we do not make an effort to articulate a substantive vision of human flourishing and instead rest the morality of our actions on the ideology of choice, we create a dangerous vacuum of moral language. Our preoccupation with choice can lead our choices to become very shallow, unexamined, and driven by larger social forces, such as the pressures of consumerism (including the pressure to buy one's way out of a problem or even the pressure to create a "better" child) or the pressures of pronatalism, which is the idea, historically more relevant to women, that to be a complete and fulfilled adult you must be a parent.

Cahill suggests that "free" choices, like the choice to be an egg donor or egg recipient, need to be examined with an awareness of the larger social context, including social structures that have historically worked to the disadvantage of women. So, whether we accept her vision of human flourishing as a test for ART or reject her disapproval of third-party donors, she raises a legitimate point about our inattention to the larger social context of "private" decisions to use ART. We need a broader, more critical discussion about the "final values or ends for which reproductive clients act."[90] Otherwise, we may discover that our free choices were not so free after all.

Summary of Key Questions

The question of moral agency: Delayed childbearing increases women's likelihood of encountering fertility problems, yet many working women today choose to delay childbearing as an adaptive strategy. Delaying childbearing is adaptive in the sense that it conforms to rather than transforms existing structures and expectations with regard to work and family, but it is purposeful in that it actively seeks the fulfillment of many legitimate life goals. Life-course decisions, such as when to have a baby, may be one of the most highly scripted in our society, but individuals subjectively understand those decisions as well. How does ART express individual agency?

The question of social justice: ART may serve economic and political interests in contradiction to the well-being of individual users, however self-aware and conscious their choices may be. We must then ask who wields the power of this technology and to what ends. Insofar as women wield the power of ART and use it to actualize their reproductive goals, who is left out of this benefit? How does ART affect existing racial and socioeconomic inequalities? Insofar as women do not wield the power of ART and its use contradicts their best interests, including potentially bodily health, what compels them to try it? Is it the promise of having it all, of combining the goals of work and family, of attaining sexual equality? Is it even appropriate to speak of "women's best interests" as a collective? What other issues of social justice are implicated in the use of ART?

The question of family goods: Families have assumed many shapes and sizes in different cultures and time periods, and the United States today witnesses a great variety of family forms. This diversity does not preclude the identification of certain goods that occur in families, including what individual family members provide for each other and how they understand the nature of their relationships and the bases of their obligations to each other. Other possible goods include what families contribute to the larger society and to future generations. Do family goods necessarily depend on having biological ties to one's children or even on having children at all? How does the use of ART impact these goods? Does ART alter parental attitudes toward children, increasing their commodification?

The Social Phenomenon of ART: Engaging the Particular

I have described selected theoretical perspectives from within feminism and Christian ethics as a way of locating some of my normative commitments and assumptions. I have also provided this account to show the inadequacy of existing theory. Cahill writes that what is "shared" in normative ethics "is not achieved beyond or over against particularity, but rather in and through it. . . . Participants in communication, judgment, and action will always be irreducibly concrete and historical characters who recognize humanity in one another, without leaving their own individuality behind."[91] Yet despite this claim's appeal, none of the ethicists I have engaged here attend seriously and consistently to the particular experience of using ART.

Donchin wisely argues that responsible ethics requires holding the general and the particular in some kind of healthy tension. I agree that it is politically naive to assume an individual woman's actions can be assessed in isolation from her social context. Likewise, it does not advance the insights of theory to assume that the general experience of a common oppression qualifies someone to judge the actions and choices of other individuals.

I have concerns about the use of ART, yet I still deeply value the resolution these technologies can offer individuals suffering from infertility. These commitments often seem to pull in opposite directions. On the one hand, an argument for social reform that might lessen the demand for ART tends to be insensitive to individual needs and individual suffering. On the other hand, attending only to individual needs and the expression of procreative liberty tends to ignore the larger impact of these technologies and the social inequalities that might be exacerbated by the growing use of ART. This book's unique methodological challenge involves holding these competing commitments together by investigating how decision making is socially shaped and how individual women experience the social practice of ART.

One primary weakness of the ethical theory discussed in previous sections is that it does not speak from experience. Feminists and religious ethicists share a tendency to focus on the general rather than the particular. They address the use of ART only in the aggregate, without verifying or testing assumptions against the diversity of people's experience with infertility. They also tend to speak on behalf of the infertile, speculating about their needs and interests.

As Barbara Berg writes in "Listening to the Voices of the Infertile," feminists have overwhelmingly approached the issue of ART from a generalized perspective:

> Feminists have entered this discussion voicing concern over the pervasive influence of pronatalism in our society, the increasing medicalization of reproduction, the commodification of women and children, the overvaluation of genetic versus social linkages, and the potential exploitation of women. There is much to be concerned about. But much of the feminist discourse on this subject has come from the perspective that these technologies should not be pursued because of their potentially negative effects on women and children. Although many legitimate concerns have been raised, complex issues have sometimes been oversimplified and, most disturbing of all, some feminists do not appear to be taking the role of advocating for infertile women so much as speaking for them. But the infertile have their own voices.[92]

It is important not to accept uncritically what these voices have to say but rather to consult and learn from them and discover where theoretical orientations were inadequate to the task of interpreting the use of ART.

The same criticism could be made of scholars in philosophical and religious ethics, including Cahill, who do not often test their normative arguments against reality. How do parents feel toward their child born of a third-party donor? Does it disrupt the parent-child relationship in the way that ethicists assumed it would? How does it affect the child's sense of identity and connection to his/her heritage? These questions cannot be answered without consulting reality, primarily because they exist at the level of interpersonal experience and individual attitudes. Similarly, do husbands or a patriarchal medical establishment pressure women to use ART? Is husband or wife more motivated to use ART, and why? If women do experience pressure to use ART, where does this pressure originate? Ethics itself cannot answer these questions but requires the input of the social sciences to devise answers and to build responsible ethical arguments that attend to the complexity of lived experience.

For all these reasons, I decided to conduct a year of empirical research, engaging in participant observation and conducting interviews with individuals experiencing infertility. In the next chapter, I introduce and describe the group I studied, RESOLVE, a national organization with a thriving Atlanta chapter.

TWO

RESOLVE

An Advocate and Forum
for the Infertile

Introduction

Once a month from September 2000 to May 2001, I observed a handful of couples and a few individuals as they gathered in the basement-level auditorium of a well-furnished Atlanta-area hospital.[1] It was fitting that the meetings occurred monthly, as the lives of most of the attendees were in many ways organized around the monthly cycles of the women there. The wait for the success or failure of an in vitro fertilization (IVF) cycle or other reproductive intervention involved what was commonly termed the "emotional roller coaster of infertility": eager hopefulness at the anticipation of pregnancy and then, more often than not, despair at the arrival of normal menstruation or the plummeting human chorionic gonadotrophin (hCG) levels[2] that signal the onset of an unstoppable miscarriage.

The women and men who came to these meetings were members of RESOLVE, a national organization founded in 1974 that supports people experiencing infertility. The organization, which has more than fifty chapters around the country, communicates an unconditional support for the resolution of infertility through one of three ways: the use of assisted reproductive technologies (now referred to by RESOLVE as "advanced reproductive technologies"), the adoption of a child or children, or the decision to remain "child-free." However, few if any of the people who came to the monthly RESOLVE meetings had not tried or were not considering some form of infertility treatment, which can range from the relatively low-tech intrauterine inseminations to the more invasive IVF.[3] Describing it as something of a rite of passage, many members spoke about the need to go through infertility treatments to grieve the loss of the experience of pregnancy and the hoped-for biological child before they felt able to consider adoption or remaining child-free. As an organizational leader said at a February 2001 session on "Transitioning from Infertility to Adoption," which was part of an annual adoption symposium sponsored by RESOLVE, "Everyone is different. Some people need to do one IVF, others need to do ten or more before they feel done. You can't rush the grieving process."[4]

Among the people for whom reproductive technologies produced a pregnancy carried to term and resulting in a live birth (statistics vary significantly according to age of the woman, but the overall average is roughly one in four), those who returned to RESOLVE meetings to share their experiences with others reported being changed permanently by the infertility experience. These women volunteers, now with children of their own, claimed no longer to be the same people they had been. Regardless of how much they formerly felt excluded from the "big club" of the "fertile world," they maintained that they still did not want to join that club and instead devoted generous amounts of time to RESOLVE.[5]

Since its founding, RESOLVE has grown to include a database of more than forty thousand individual members and providers of infertility services.[6] In addition to an active and loyal membership base, RESOLVE has developed a prominent voice as a public advocate for the infertile and is widely cited in the popular media and bioethics literature. Its reach is broad and its reputation well known. According to RESOLVE's national Web site, the national office and local chapters handle some 1.5 million contacts per year from people looking for information about infertility.[7] Among people I have met who are experiencing or who have experienced infertility, most have at least heard of RESOLVE, even if they have not chosen to join.

Although RESOLVE identifies itself as a loyal advocate for the interests of the infertile, RESOLVE's membership by no means fully represents everyone who has fertility problems. Based on my observations at the time I conducted my research, RESOLVE's membership mirrored the demographic picture of people who use assisted reproductive technologies (ART): married, middle or upper-middle class, and largely white. However, RESOLVE's official policy is one of inclusion: "In principle and in practice, RESOLVE seeks a diverse membership. There shall be no barrier to full participation in this organization."[8] How and why RESOLVE serves this particular demographic group is an open question but probably has a great deal to do with the perceived fit between the organization's values and those of the individuals seeking to overcome their infertility. As with any institution in our diverse society, RESOLVE likely draws people who self-select based on their perception of how well the organization will meet their needs.

For many reasons, my choice of RESOLVE as the central focus of my field research entailed some obvious limitations. RESOLVE is only one group, and although its size and geographic reach make it a significant group, it cannot represent the full range of the infertility experience in the United States. Insofar as RESOLVE presents a limited view of the infertility experience, so too will my reporting of the infertility experience be limited. Within RESOLVE, I focused more narrowly still on one local chapter, which happened to be located in Atlanta. (See appendix A for my reasons for choosing RESOLVE and for focusing on a single group.)

A National Organization and a Local Community

Mission and Structure

One of RESOLVE's stated commitments, printed as a motto on almost all of the group's documents, is "to provide timely, compassionate support and information to people who are experiencing infertility and to increase awareness of infertility issues through public education and advocacy." In the organizational division of labor that seems characteristic of RESOLVE, the national office (which members commonly refer to as "national") tends mainly to the latter half of this mission, especially to advocacy on a national level, while the local chapters tend to the provision of support and information in face-to-face interactions. One benefit of this two-part structure is that it allows rigorous advocacy on behalf of the infertile, primarily in the form of congressional lobbying and the annual National Infertility Awareness Week, without necessarily draining the emotional resources of people who seek the support of RESOLVE on the local level. There is almost a sense in which the local chapters care for the currently wounded while the national office is the outlet of the healed—those who have survived infertility and have gone on to make education, support, and advocacy on behalf of the infertile their life's work.

The National Level

The national headquarters, historically located in Somerville, Massachusetts, but moved to Bethesda, Maryland, in November 2004, has paid staff, financial supporters, a newsletter, and a Web site. The group's greatest stated priority is supporting the interests of the infertile. But how are those interests defined?

One of RESOLVE's main agendas, easily discerned from the national newsletter or the "Advocacy Action" e-mail updates that members receive, is insurance coverage for infertility treatments. RESOLVE lobbies for legislative changes that would mandate insurance coverage for all diagnostic procedures and infertility treatments. Key to the group's justification for coverage is the argument that infertility should be considered an illness or disease and therefore treated the same as any other illness or disease.

As of 2004, fifteen states had enacted some form of infertility insurance mandate, with Massachusetts the most generous.[9] RESOLVE credits the grassroots efforts of its volunteers and the American Society of Reproductive Medicine (ASRM) with achieving this legislation.[10] At the time of my research, "Advocacy Action" updates described other legislation that RESOLVE strongly supported. One example was the Family Building Act of 2001, which required health plans to cover infertility treatments and defined infertility as a disease requiring care, just like other medical conditions. RESOLVE also supported the Fair Access to Infertility Treatment and Hope (FAITH) Act of 2001, which required coverage of infertility treatments in all health insurance plans. According to RESOLVE, "The FAITH Act will limit the number of infertility treatment cycles to four, and would include procedures deemed appropriate by the physician and patient such as drug therapy, artificial insemination, in vitro fertilization (IVF), and embryo donation. According to insurance industry estimates, this legislation would have minimal effect on the cost of health insurance, increasing the cost by as little as 21 cents per month per person."[11] To my knowledge, neither bill became law.

Outside of RESOLVE, debate continues over whether mandated insurance coverage for infertility treatment is appropriate or fair. It is by no means a foregone conclusion that people are entitled to positive assistance in their efforts to reproduce. Moreover, as with all medical treatments in an era of managed care, infertility treatments are subjected to cost-benefit analysis and the scrutiny that comes with trying to determine the legitimacy and priority of a given treatment when not all treatments can be covered. Estimates about the cost of covering infertility treatments vary greatly, making judgment difficult. In contrast with the FAITH bill's claims that the increased costs of covering ART would be minimal, one group complying with a legislated insurance mandate emphasizes a high cost for the small number served: "The Massachusetts Association of Health Maintenance Organizations says its members pay $40 million more in premiums to cover infertility treatment for 2000 couples."[12]

Yet RESOLVE publications take an unequivocal stand that full insurance coverage is appropriate. A national RESOLVE briefing paper, *Infertility and Insurance Coverage*, assesses general attitudes toward treating infertility as an illness and makes clear the group's position: "While public awareness of infertility has increased in the last decade, public policymakers, employers and insurance companies have been slow to recognize infertility as a legitimate medical problem."[13] The publication then explains why infertility should be considered a legitimate medical problem. For one, the origins of infertility resemble other major illnesses: infertility almost always has some physiological cause or causes, and medical advances now enable the identification of these underlying problems with unprecedented accuracy. According to RESOLVE, roughly 40 percent of cases of infertility result from female infertility problems, 40 percent result from male infertility problems, 10 percent result from combined male and female factors, and 10 percent are idiopathic or unexplained.[14] In addition, the effects or consequences of infertility resemble other major illnesses: the inability to reproduce can be devastating emotionally and psychologically. Studies have shown that anxiety and depression levels in women with infertility resemble those of women with cancer, hypertension, heart disease, or HIV.

Beyond these claims, the briefing paper points to what may be special about reproductive activity, arguing that procreation is a fundamental human right and that society is thus obligated to provide access to health services for the treatment of infertility. Appealing to legal precedent, the briefing paper identifies reproduction as a "major life activity" that warrants protection from discrimination through the Americans with Disabilities Act. Thus, denying insurance coverage for infertility treatments but providing it for prenatal checkups and a postpartum hospital room, for example, might be discriminatory. Finally, *Infertility and Insurance Coverage* argues that insurance coverage is warranted because infertility treatments are not experimental, reasoning that (1) the ASRM and the American College of Obstetricians and Gynecologists no longer classify infertility treatments as experimental and (2) tens of thousands of babies have been born from ART.[15] For all of these reasons, the briefing paper concludes that infertility warrants the same compassion and treatment that other diseases and illnesses receive, including insurance coverage.

As for concerns about fairness, which the briefing paper on insurance coverage also addresses, RESOLVE supplies evidence that infertility treatments are not too costly for society to bear. On a national scale, the total spent on infertility treatments in 1996 was $2.6 billion, only a "tiny fraction" (roughly 0.25 percent) of the total U.S. health care budget. In response to those who might point to the millions of uninsured in this country who lack access to any health care as reason to limit coverage for infertility treatments, RESOLVE acknowledges the seriousness of the problem but argues that it is unfair for premiums paid by infertile people to help cover maternity benefits for the fertile when coverage for infertility treatments is not provided. Those who have health insurance coverage ought to be able to access the health care services they need, RESOLVE argues.

Although lobbying for insurance coverage of infertility treatments is a major agenda of the national RESOLVE office, it is not the only agenda. RESOLVE also strongly supports making adoption a more accessible option for infertile couples. In 2001, RESOLVE attained one of its major goals, an increased adoption tax credit, with the passage of the Hope for Children Act, which increased the credit from five thousand dollars to ten thousand dollars per child for qualified expenses and gave a flat ten thousand dollars for special needs without regard to expenses.[16]

RESOLVE also supports the prevention of sexually transmitted diseases, which can cause infertility if left untreated. For example, RESOLVE helped to publicize efforts by the Center for Health and Gender Equity to advocate increased government support of the development of microbicides, topical agents that prevent the transmission of sexually transmitted diseases. RESOLVE also vocally supports the Family and Medical Leave Act, primarily because it allows time off from work for a "serious health condition" (including infertility) and its treatment and for the birth or adoption of a child.[17]

Other issues are less prominent on or even absent from the national RESOLVE agenda. For example, robust advocacy for legislation that would regulate clinics, including the practices of egg and sperm donation, does not seem to be a high priority. Compared with the energy and space given to the insurance coverage issue, little attention is paid to the improvement of the safety of procedures and drugs used in infertility treatment, especially more experimental procedures such as intracytoplasmic sperm injection, which proceeded to human use without extensive research trials in other mammals, or cytoplasmic transfer, which animal studies have shown produces offspring with genetic mutations.[18] Neither RESOLVE's national Web site nor the group's book, *Resolving Infertility: Understanding the Options and Choosing Solutions When You Want to Have a Baby* (1999), offers specific information about safety.

The Fertility Clinic Success Rate and Certification Act of 1992 is the only federal statute that directly regulates assisted reproduction. The act requires that the Centers for Disease Control annually collect data about the success rates of U.S. ART clinics and make that information public to consumers. This collection of data, known as the ART Report, is available online. Each clinic is required to disclose its success rates (take-home baby rates) for all of the various types of ART offered as well as "failure rates" (no pregnancy was detected) and rates of miscarriage and ectopic pregnancy. The information is further broken down by factors such as age of patient, whether fresh or frozen sperm were used, and whether donor or patient eggs were used. The Fertility Clinic Success Rate and Certification Act also includes an entirely voluntary set of standards that states can use if they choose to require their embryo laboratories to be certified and want to ensure consistent quality control.[19]

Because the U.S. Food and Drug Administration (FDA) has no jurisdiction over the practice of medicine, there is no direct federal oversight of physicians who provide infertility services. Monitoring the competent and ethical practice of medicine has always been left to the states, largely through licensure requirements. Thus, state-level regulation of ART occurs indirectly, through the regulation of medicine generally.[20] A few states have enacted laws that directly regulate the provision and consumption of ART, but most have not. The majority of existing state laws that attempt to regulate ART instead address issues of access and insurance coverage.[21]

Insofar as the FDA has any regulatory power over ART, it is limited to the approval of new drugs. However, physicians are generally permitted to use drugs in novel ways without obtaining additional approval from the FDA as long as the drugs have been approved for their originally intended purpose. Such "off-label" use falls under the legitimate practice of medicine, which lies beyond the FDA's authority. Many of the drugs used during an IVF cycle were originally approved for other purposes. For example, Lupron, which suppresses ovulation during an IVF cycle, was originally approved to treat endometriosis and uterine fibroids.[22] Moreover, sperm, eggs, and embryos are not classified as drugs that can be regulated, and categorizing them as drugs would make little sense.[23]

Significantly, given this context of arguably limited or piecemeal regulation, RESOLVE views the current regulation of the infertility industry in the United States as basically adequate: "RESOLVE supports uniform regulations, standards, and guidelines that protect the integrity of prospective parents and donors, their gametes, and any resulting children but which do not limit access to medically appropriate treatment."[24] The group consistently emphasizes access. In press releases and official publications, national RESOLVE seems at least as invested in maximizing patients' treatment options as it is in scrutinizing or regulating ART. RESOLVE certainly endorses the main function of the ART Report, which is to hold clinics accountable by publicizing details of their practices and providing a useful caveat emptor to prospective patients. Indeed, prior to 2004, RESOLVE served as one of the ART Report's coauthors, along with the Centers for Disease Control, the ASRM, and the Society for Assisted Reproductive Technology. However, RESOLVE is no longer listed as a coauthor of the ART Report because the group now comments on the report from the consumer perspective.[25] RESOLVE also now insists that the pressure of publishing success rates has had the unwanted side effect of barring some patients with lower chances of success from receiving treatment.[26]

Concerns about the long-term effects of ART do not receive the same prominent attention afforded insurance coverage and access. I have neither heard RESOLVE officials mention nor read in the group's publications any support for the rights of children born through these procedures (for example, for the right to access medical information about gamete donors). The group also devotes little attention to the importance of disclosing risks of cancer and other future health problems for women and the children born through ART beyond basic support for informed consent. Also absent from the national agenda is a discussion of the problem of women who encounter difficulty in obtaining health insurance after undergoing infertility treatments.[27] It is possible that health insurance actuaries have information about the long-term health risks of infertility treatments of which the general public may not be aware and which RESOLVE's public education efforts do not necessarily foreground.

The Local Level

RESOLVE includes some fifty chapters around the country, all of which have close ties to the national office. Membership dues are split evenly between the national office and the local chapters. Meetings and conferences keep local chapter leaders in contact with national, and each local chapter provides basically the same membership services: meetings, support groups, telephone help lines, newsletters, and referrals.

The local chapter that I studied, RESOLVE of Georgia, is one of the country's ten largest chapters. It is a vibrant organization with many active participants. The monthly meetings were always well attended and seemed to be the core from which other chapter activities radiated. Members could attend the meetings for free, while nonmembers paid $10 to attend. Numerous volunteers ran the monthly meetings and the other chapter activities, including several peer-led "living room discussion groups" and therapist-led support groups around the metro Atlanta area. Only members could attend these sessions. Other services included physician referrals, member-to-member contacts, a medical information service, and the *RESOLVE of Georgia Newsletter*, which I received during the year I conducted my research. The newsletter included articles by RESOLVE members from around the country and often reprinted popular articles that had appeared previously. It also published informational articles by local physicians and current announcements about legislative victories, leadership changes, and local events. Roughly half the pages of the *RESOLVE of Georgia Newsletter* at the time of my research were paid advertisements—at a cost of $250 for a full-page ad—from area fertility clinics, drug companies, local pharmacies, adoption agencies, adoption attorneys, and the Internet company IVF.com.

I observed ten monthly meetings and two all-day Saturday symposia during the 2000–2001 program year. I also interviewed individual members and RESOLVE leaders as I became more familiar with the group. At the beginning of my research, I asked to attend one of the peer-led or therapist-led support groups, where I hoped to encounter a more consistent group of individuals, but was denied permission because RESOLVE leaders believed that the presence of an outside observer would be detrimental to the group's dynamics and participants' comfort level. The women who made the decision conveyed a strong sense of protectiveness about group members' vulnerabilities.

It quickly became apparent, however, that the monthly public meetings provided an excellent site for field research. There was a remarkable consistency in the people who attended, the discussions were interesting and candid, and the presentations were highly informative. Since the meetings were public, theoretically anyone could come and ask questions and participate. However, the meetings rarely strayed from the kinds of discussions and question-and-answer periods that members found acceptable.

Each monthly meeting had a different focus, and most involved an outside speaker or speakers. Chapter leaders, who were in regular contact with national officials, selected the topics in accordance with members' needs, providing information about various types of ART and adoption and providing support for dealing with infertility in the context of a wider life. Topics of the meetings I attended included "Ask the Experts" (an informational medical symposium with several local physicians), "Coping with the Holidays" (with a presentation by a psychotherapist), "Navigating the Infertility Information Highway" (with a presentation by the owner of IVF.com), "The Medical, Financial, Legal, and Emotional Aspects of Using Donor Egg or Sperm or Surrogate" (with presentations by a physician, psychologist, attorney, and financial adviser), and "Disclosure: How Do We Tell Our Child/Children?" (with a presentation by a woman who had used an egg donor to conceive her daughter and a discussion facilitated by a long-time RESOLVE member and national leader). (See table A.1 for a complete list of 2000–2001 monthly meeting topics.)

I also attended a February 2001 adoption symposium, which offered information about domestic, international, and special-needs adoptions; the legal aspects of adoption; preparing for home study; and the psychological aspects of parenting after adoption, among other topics.

The group was considering some new topics for the 2001–2 program year, after my research concluded, including "Women, Infertility, and Body Image" and "Resolutions: When Enough Is Enough . . . Moving On." Also new for that year was a monthly meeting focused solely on adoption, to be held in addition to the annual all-day Saturday symposium on adoption.

All monthly meetings followed a pattern. The first hour was an informal "peer-led" or "member-to-member" discussion, which ran like a support group. The second hour and a half or more was set aside for a panel presentation or other formal presentation by the outside speaker or speakers. This second part tended to be more informational but, depending on who was giving the presentation, could also provide another opportunity for informal discussion. For example, when physicians addressed the group, the presentations were more formal and all questions were held to the end. When therapists addressed the group, in contrast, the presentations were more like facilitated discussions, often continuing conversations started in the earlier part of the meeting. Both parts of the meeting usually took place in the basement-level hospital auditorium with everyone sitting in rows in cushioned theater seats. On a few occasions, the peer discussion was held in a smaller classroom next door, with metal chairs arranged in a circle.[28] Most people attended meetings in their entirety, but a few people arrived late and attended only the more informational part of the meeting.

At the end of the meetings I attended, it was common for one of the chapter copresidents, an energetic and cheerful native southerner who was the mother of two children through IVF, to admonish the attendees, "Don't leave here tonight without talking to at least one other person." Having reached the "other side" of infertility, she spoke with an earnest, compassionate, and hopeful voice. She often explained that the monthly meetings sought to provide a place where people could "connect" because infertility can be an isolating experience. Meetings also enabled people to "feel normal" and to meet others "going through the same thing you are." While the copresident said that she and the other RESOLVE leaders and organizers worked hard to provide meetings that were full of relevant technical and medical information (as at the "Ask the Experts" meeting, which included six Atlanta-area specialists in reproductive medicine), she stated to the group her belief that members can and do get a lot of that information elsewhere. She saw emotional support as RESOLVE's primary mission, at least at the local level.

She reiterated these themes in an interview, deemphasizing RESOLVE's need to provide content-specific information or to attract a certain number of attendees and highlighting RESOLVE's responsibility to provide a forum for discussion and connection, a responsibility she likened to a mission: "The numbers aren't really that important. What is important to me is that these couples meet another couple. That they connect. Because so many times people come in, they listen, they walk out and, yeah, they got the information, but if you don't meet somebody else that's going through it, you still feel isolated and like you're still alone in this. So, for me, it's been for us to provide a forum for them to get to know other couples. And it's not as important what information we provide, as much as the people they get to meet."[29] This emphasis on personal connection distinguished local RESOLVE from national RESOLVE. Under the rubric of experiencing infertility, the local RESOLVE meetings brought together individuals who might not otherwise find each other. The group brought together sufferers and provided a space in which they could support each other. But this forum was not devoid of content. It was not without agendas. In many respects, large and small, the local meetings followed the national organization's mission.

RESOLVE'S Self-Understanding

A Neutral Forum?

In keeping with the national office's public statements, RESOLVE of Georgia saw itself as providing unconditional support to people facing infertility. RESOLVE generally sees itself as being neutral or nonjudgmental about major aspects of infertility, especially about how to resolve it. In what follows, I will provide some evidence of this self-understanding and then begin to critique it based on what may be RESOLVE's most important work, redefining and reframing key terms and aspects of the infertility experience and its resolution, work that is decidedly moral (that is, nonneutral) in its mission.

Many spoken and written statements indicate that RESOLVE sees itself as providing a neutral space for its members. Perhaps most notable is the organization's official statement on what it terms "family building": "RESOLVE supports family-building through a variety of methods, including appropriate medical treatment, adoption, surrogacy and the choice of childfree living."[30] Consistent with this position, the local chapter endeavored to convey the sense that all options for resolving infertility are equally valid. Although not every option received equal time and attention at monthly meetings, all options were discussed respectfully and seriously when they arose. No choice was labeled, at least explicitly, out of bounds. In addition, the experiences of the volunteers who organized and spoke at the monthly meetings embodied the different paths to resolving infertility: roughly comparable numbers of female volunteers had borne children through ART and had adopted, and a smaller number of volunteers and group leaders were living "child-free." None of the local chapter's volunteers, to my knowledge, had used surrogacy.[31]

A similar example of providing neutral space—in this case, written space—involved the local newsletter. Like the national newsletter, which accepts financial sponsorship from many fertility clinics around the country to support its publication but states that "sponsorship does not constitute endorsement by

RESOLVE," RESOLVE of Georgia had a policy of nonendorsement of all products and services advertised in its quarterly newsletter and nonendorsement of the views expressed in that newsletter. As a result, for example, at one monthly meeting, the guest speaker—an Atlanta-area physician with a Web site and chat room in which he answers questions about infertility—expressed disagreement with an ASRM statement, reprinted in the *RESOLVE of Georgia Newsletter*, that shared-risk programs for in vitro fertilization were ethically problematic.[32] When the speaker finished defending the virtues of shared-risk programs and expressing his disapproval of the newsletter article, the copresident of the local chapter, who had been sitting in the front row, stood up and clarified that only ASRM, not RESOLVE, had criticized the shared-risk programs. She emphasized that RESOLVE does not necessarily endorse the views of the articles published in its newsletter.

The newsletter's neutrality mirrored that of the public space of monthly meetings. On occasion, leaders asked participants not to "doctor bash" during meetings, because these statements could find their way back to area clinics, which would then hold RESOLVE responsible. Similarly, when someone tried to solicit a judgment about a particular physician at a meeting, she was told that RESOLVE does not make evaluative statements about local clinics or physicians. With membership in RESOLVE of Georgia comes a referral list, several pages long, of physicians in the southern region, but the group makes no specific recommendations.

This self-understanding of neutrality, of not taking critical positions on providers or practices, extended beyond specific policies about what could be said at meetings or printed in newsletters. In a larger sense, RESOLVE sees itself as providing something that no other institution in our society can provide. In an article, "The Value of a Non-Profit in a Changing World," RESOLVE executive director Diane Aronson explicitly described the group's self-perception: "With the changes in the field, the growing value of RESOLVE remains in the fact that we provide unbiased information and support—an oasis of clear guidance, with no strings attached, a haven of trust within a confine of competition and information overload."[33] This statement articulates a vision of the organization as above the fray, as beyond the compromising pressures of the market, and as qualitatively different from other institutions in a "changing world." As a nonprofit, RESOLVE can credibly portray itself as educating and supporting rather than selling or persuading.

Although RESOLVE clearly extends considerable loyalty to the medical establishment, it is equally clear that medical professionals and fertility clinics are not in a position to support people experiencing infertility the way

RESOLVE believes it can. A national RESOLVE newsletter article advised people experiencing infertility about how to navigate today's medical world:

> Though these miraculous technologies are now available, the reality of the business nature of medicine has made it necessary for consumers to be more scrutinizing of the medical team. . . . It is essential that you be an informed consumer. . . . Most infertility consumers are not schooled in medicine, so the staff should understand your need to hear information about complex procedures repeated more than once. . . . The available options for infertility treatment have expanded significantly over the years. This good news is accompanied by the added responsibility of needing to be a wise consumer. Today's medical environment is a different world from the one our parents experienced. Today, the health care consumer is part of the team.[34]

The article offers the sound advice that with added choice comes added responsibility by distancing itself somewhat from without openly criticizing the "business nature" of medicine. The reader gets an image of RESOLVE as taking the side of the individual infertile patient and encouraging the patient to be a wise consumer.

If RESOLVE sees itself as distinct from the business-oriented medical establishment, it also sees itself as distinct from religion and religious institutions, which apply distinct pressures to individuals deciding which infertility treatments to try. A *RESOLVE of Georgia Newsletter* article presents a contrasting picture of what religion and RESOLVE can offer people experiencing infertility: "Religion and philosophy provide a reflective and ethical approach to the use of new reproductive technologies, which are in themselves often morally neutral. . . . Religions can reinvigorate family building activities and there is an important place for them in the infertility, adoption, and child free worlds." However, for its part, "RESOLVE compassionately cares for those facing family building options and supports knowledge of options being accessible."[35] Chapter 3 will present a more in-depth discussion of RESOLVE's view of and relationship to religion and ethics, but I note here that the organization takes great care to portray itself as open-minded and compassionate. Its role is not to judge or even necessarily to question but to support unconditionally individuals' choices from an array of ostensibly neutral options.

Ultimately, rather than saying that the group is truly neutral or believes itself to be neutral, a more accurate assessment of the organization's self-perception may be that it tolerates a diverse range of experiences and points of view for the greater good of hope. For at least two years, RESOLVE of Georgia commenced its monthly meetings in September with the same theme:

"The Many Faces of RESOLVE, The Many Reasons for Hope." At the September 2000 celebration of the twentieth anniversary of the founding of RESOLVE of Georgia, the speakers—founders and former leaders, including some who had gone on to positions in the national organization—testified to the different approaches and different experiences that underlie the common hope for a "life after infertility."[36]

The Work of Redefinition

Despite the rhetoric of neutrality, I believe that RESOLVE actively works to redefine or reframe the experience of infertility and that this work of redefinition is central to its mission of offering support. While the larger society may define or label infertility in ways that are stigmatizing and unsupportive of individuals, RESOLVE works to transform these definitions and perceptions into something more tolerant, hopeful, and compassionate. Moreover, these implicit moral values are already present in RESOLVE's commitment to neutrality or being "unbiased." RESOLVE's literature, including pamphlets for members and informational fact sheets, offer numerous examples of this ongoing work of redefinition, including how the biases and assumptions of the "fertile world" are challenged and transformed by the "infertile world."

Language is powerful, and the words used to describe an experience can have tremendous impact on how the experience is processed and the meaning that it is given. Inside RESOLVE, infertility is defined as a legitimate illness, the goal of having children is called "family building" rather than "starting a family," and the meaning of "resolving infertility" includes adoption and choosing to remain "child-free."

Outside of RESOLVE, the medical establishment has a notorious history of perpetuating language that imparts a sense of guilt, inadequacy, and/or powerlessness, particularly to women experiencing reproductive problems. Examples of such terminology include an "incompetent cervix" (cervix that tends to dilate prematurely during pregnancy), "premature ovarian failure" (early menopause), "elderly prima gravida" (a woman pregnant for the first time at age thirty-five or older), "habitual aborter" (a woman who tends to have recurring, spontaneous miscarriages), and the archaic-sounding "expected date of confinement" (due date for childbirth).[37] Terms such as "failure" and "incompetent" are not often seen in conjunction with male-factor infertility. A varicose vein around the testes that can cause infertility is simply called a varicocele, not testicular failure. A low number of healthy, motile sperm is simply a low sperm count, not incompetent sperm.

The literature of RESOLVE leads by example, using more neutral terms to describe medical conditions and taking great care not to impart guilt or responsibility for infertility. Like other women's health groups born in the 1960s and 1970s, including the Boston Women's Health Book Collective, RESOLVE was influenced by the social movement to advocate for patients' interests.[38] The work of redefinition grew out of the movement to obtain more rights and power for patients and to challenge medical professionals' paternalistic authority. However, RESOLVE's work expands beyond the feminist goals of criticizing medical terms perceived as demeaning to women.[39] Indeed, RESOLVE is decidedly not interested in antagonizing the medical establishment but rather seeks to challenge and transform society's tendency to stigmatize infertility and the people—both women and men—who suffer from it.

RESOLVE's work, including its work of redefinition, has thus become more mainstream. The medical establishment offers an important legitimacy to the diagnosis and treatment of infertility and is therefore not to be treated as the enemy. This friendlier relationship with the medical establishment is one of the things that distinguishes RESOLVE from older grassroots women's health groups, like the Boston Women's Health Book Collective, which tended instead to cultivate ties with progressive or radical social movements. Sheryl Ruzek describes some other differences between what she calls more professionalized mainstream organizations, of which RESOLVE may be a good example, and grassroots women's health movement groups. The professionalized support and advocacy groups born in the 1990s tend to be more narrowly focused on a single disease or health issue and draw their leadership from highly trained professionals rather than laypersons. Some other differences include the fact that older feminist groups focused on the need to protect women from unsafe medical interventions, whereas the newer groups focus more on ensuring women equitable access to advances in biotechnology and treatment. And while older feminist groups tended to distance themselves from corporate sponsors, fearing that these financial ties might compromise their ability to criticize such companies or promote alternative therapies, newer groups rely heavily on corporate sponsorship.[40]

RESOLVE unquestionably relies on corporate sponsorship. Each monthly meeting typically had at least one corporate sponsor (for example, a pharmaceutical company). The national RESOLVE Web site also facilitates a dialogue between consumers and the infertility industry through its Corporate Council, which provides a "forum for members of the industry with products and services of interest to individuals dealing with infertility to have a significant dialog with RESOLVE regarding the strategic direction and objectives for research, education, and advocacy for family building issues." The list of industry members on RESOLVE's Corporate Council includes Ferring Pharmaceuticals, Gynecare, IntegraMed America, ivpcare, Organon, Repromedix, Serono, ViaCyte, and Village Pharmacy.[41]

RESOLVE's relationship with the infertility industry does not negate the work of redefinition on either the local or national level. However, it would be myopic not to situate RESOLVE's ambitions and goals in the larger context in which they are pursued, which includes a complicated relationship with those who stand to profit substantially from the consumption of infertility services. Potential costs and benefits arise when operating in this context rather than in opposition to it, and it is important to bear these factors in mind as specific instances of redefinition are considered.

Infertility as Illness

By defining infertility as an illness, RESOLVE accomplishes many important tasks. This definition legitimizes the experience of infertility as real. Before advances in medicine made it possible to identify physiological causes of infertility, childlessness was understood in ways that differ dramatically from the idea of illness. People commonly (and often erroneously) believed that the inability to conceive resulted from psychological problems, such as stress or an unacknowledged rejection of pregnancy.[42] Because the various physiological causes, including female-factor, male-factor, and combined female- and male-factor infertility, were not well understood, women or their psychological conditions were often blamed for the inability to become pregnant. Many RESOLVE members take the admonition, "Just relax, you'll get pregnant," as evidence that this misperception persists.[43]

Another powerful and even older misperception that still lingers in society is that infertility is the will of God. Defining infertility as an illness removes the matter from the terminology of the theological or cosmological and places it squarely in the domain of practical medicine. RESOLVE works hard to counter the ideas, internalized by many infertile couples who seek out RESOLVE's support, that individuals are somehow to blame for their infertility; that infertility is punishment for past wrongs, such as an abortion; and that people who are infertile are somehow lesser people or less worthy of being parents. If infertility is understood as a potentially treatable illness, it becomes only a piece of an individual's experience, not the existential condition of the person as a whole. Moreover, if infertility is an illness that can yield to human medical intervention, it cannot logically be called divine punishment. It falls far short of this otherworldly condemnation. The guilt that people bring to their fertility problems can then begin to be assuaged and replaced with greater compassion.

Finally, as discussed earlier, defining infertility as an illness has the very pragmatic benefit of increasing the likelihood that infertility treatments will qualify for insurance coverage. Analogies between infertility and other major stress-inducing illnesses, such as cancer, are common in RESOLVE's literature. The legitimacy of illness thus lends legitimacy to the experience of infertility.[44]

"Family Building"

Another important example of redefinition is the term "family building," which sounds somewhat odd to the novice RESOLVE member but soon becomes standard vocabulary for everyone. All of RESOLVE's literature uses this term—the group now publishes a magazine called *Family Building*—and its definition is explicitly and frequently reiterated. "Starting a family" is considered offensive because it assumes that only children constitute the "start" of a family and implies that a committed or married couple cannot consider themselves a real family until they have a child. "Family building," by contrast, assumes that a family already exists when there are just adults: two people who are committed to each other and who consider themselves to be a family *are* a family. "Family building" simply acknowledges the desire to expand or grow in number. The term therefore also includes people experiencing secondary infertility (a couple with one child having difficulty conceiving a second). With either primary or secondary infertility, the term "family building" does not necessarily imply conception, pregnancy, and birth but can and often does mean adoption.

One notable aspect of the term "family building" is that it is also a construction metaphor, an active image of making something, and it thus draws on the same proactive, propatient assumptions present in the idea of treating and overcoming an illness. RESOLVE is by no measure an organization that embraces a fatalistic outlook on life. It counsels its members not to endure suffering and be patient with infertility but actively to work to solve the problem. Patient empowerment is among RESOLVE's most important goals, with the ultimate goal of moving completely beyond the experience of infertility.

"Resolving" Infertility

Given this goal, the organization's name and the significance of what it means to "resolve infertility" should not be overlooked. Since the birth of modern medicine, human beings have ventured to apply will and determination where nature and fate formerly controlled. The idea that one could "resolve" to overcome one's infertility carries with it certain assumptions about what lies within human power as well as about the impact of psychological orientation on infertility. The availability and considerable sophistication of ART has vastly expanded the options for people who experience infertility. Only in recent decades has it even been possible to contemplate treating infertility by circumventing the event of in vivo fertilization. But resolving infertility can also be a deliberate decision to adopt, perhaps without trying ART or trying only a few of the available technologies. Resolving infertility can also mean deciding not to pursue parenthood at all and instead enjoying what is called child-free living.

The term "child-free living" is a source of some debate within the organization. Some individuals who have chosen not to parent believe the term "child-free" falsely implies that their lives are devoid of any children. However, I take the term "child-free" as another clear example of RESOLVE's reframing: taking a lack and turning it into something positive, something embraced or deliberately chosen rather than something simply endured.

An article by Margaret Beck, director of clinical services at the Massachusetts chapter of RESOLVE, "Making the Leap to Adoption," describes infertility from firsthand experience, with special attention to what it means to "move beyond" infertility to resolution.

> During treatment, it is normal and even healthy to employ a certain level of denial, which protects you and enables you to go forward. It is important to become more realistic about the true costs, emotional, physical and financial, of treatment. It is also important to begin to look at your life in its fullness, moving beyond this one goal and remembering all your various hopes and dreams for a full, rich life. This is also a good time to take stock of all the various reasons that you continue treatment, besides the drive to have a biological child. You may find that you are continuing treatment to avoid the pain of stopping; sometimes it is too difficult to imagine the next step; or you may feel you must do "everything possible" to have done enough. Often, because you have valued hard work and sacrifice, it can be disturbing to encounter an area where hard work is ineffective. You may find that you have to reformulate the idea of stopping treatment not as "giving up," but as deeply honoring your entire self in the need to move on in life.[45]

This article hits many of the common notes of RESOLVE meetings: it begins from the assumption that the reader is undergoing treatment and expresses sympathy for and an intuitive awareness of the reasons why stopping treatment is difficult. These reasons center on the disappointment of not being able to meet goals and the unsettling inversion of the benefits of hard work. It then moves to a place where stopping treatment can be redefined and accepted.

Stopping represents not defeat or failure but a conscious decision to resume the wider activities of a full life—that is, full of goals that extend beyond the goal of parenthood.

This article also articulates, in more detail than I usually encountered in group conversations, the loss that infertility represents:

> Creating a baby is a wonderful, rich and tender dream. Babies made in love tie us to our partners powerfully and irrevocably, for all time. Babies tie us to our pasts, our parents and siblings and way beyond. They tie us to our future. Babies that we create tie us to our physical selves, as our bodies bring forth this truly awesome miracle. And, babies tie us to all human kind, since all babies are made in basically this same way. Making babies is both mundane and miraculous; to feel left out of this process represents a huge and sorrowful loss. For many of you, coming to grips with this loss is one of the biggest emotional challenges of your lives.[46]

Finally, Beck's article redefines the process of dealing with infertility, encouraging the shift from an orientation of practical problem solving and making the "right" choice to one of acceptance and optimism. She uses the example of adoption:

> It is natural to wonder how important pregnancy or genetic continuity is in the passion of your love for a child. It is natural to wonder if your child will love you as passionately, knowing that he or she has another set of parents. The answer is basic, but profound: no one can describe the transforming power of parent-child love. . . . We all have a natural tendency to think that we have to make the very most right decision about these issues and that the rest will be easy. In fact, the real challenge may actually be in living out whatever decision we have made with creativity, energy, optimism and joy. We make the "right" decision "right" by how we live it out.[47]

Later chapters will return to the example of adoption and of what "taking the leap" to adoption after infertility treatment seemed to represent for people in RESOLVE. Noteworthy in this context, however, is RESOLVE's active role in reframing the experience of infertility for its members.

While ostensibly serving as a neutral forum in which people can connect with one another on an emotional level, RESOLVE's mission is not neutral in the sense of lacking substantive moral content. At both the national and local levels, RESOLVE is committed to providing unconditional support to its members, and an important part of this support is to direct them to "resolution."

The Function(s) of the Monthly Meetings

Sharing the Infertility Journey

Since RESOLVE's overarching mission is to direct its members to the resolution of infertility, it is not surprising that its monthly meetings functioned a lot like a support group. That is, they functioned mainly to support participants' individual choices. Understanding in greater detail how these meetings functioned will help illuminate the substance of the group's values, including the extent to which RESOLVE inculcated a critical perspective toward ART, the infertility industry, or any of the conditions giving rise to the problem of infertility.

In his study, *Sharing the Journey: Support Groups and America's New Quest for Community* (1994), sociologist Robert Wuthnow describes what he calls the small-group movement—a staggering proliferation of Sunday school classes, Bible study groups, self-help groups, and special interest groups (such as book discussion groups, sports/hobby groups, and groups that discuss politics or current events). Wuthnow hypothesizes that the existence of these groups poses a challenge to recent claims that community life has been eroded in the United States at the expense of unbridled individualism. After surveying the landscape of small groups in this country and investigating what takes place during their meetings, however, he concludes that they do not necessarily mitigate our individualistic tendencies. People still come to these groups to work on their individual goals and problems but do so in the company of others. As Ann Swidler summarizes, "These groups offer more of the same kind of community Americans have always built—groups that serve individual aims and affirm the self, and yet make no onerous, enduring demands."[48]

Of the types of small groups Wuthnow studied, I believe RESOLVE is most like a self-help group in structure (composed of peers who share common experiences), demographics (largely white), and purpose (to provide emotional support), although RESOLVE lacks a specifically Christian orientation. RESOLVE does not have an explicit religious affiliation and understands itself to be "open to the masses." RESOLVE meetings were not, however, without significant spiritual dimensions and concerns. "Coming to grips" with the "huge and sorrowful loss" that infertility represents tended to raise spiritual issues, which were discussed openly during the monthly meetings. One notable difference between RESOLVE monthly meetings and the small groups described by Wuthnow is that RESOLVE members tend to join for longer than typical small-group members. Indeed, the loyalty of RESOLVE members at the local level, even after resolving their infertility, was striking.

The strength of this feeling of affiliation and membership suggests that the role of individualism in small groups may be more ambiguous than Wuthnow concludes. On the one hand, only the purportedly individualistic aim of having a child brings RESOLVE members together. On the other hand, in many cases, the community of RESOLVE seems to outlast the accomplishment of this goal. What is the significance of this phenomenon? What are the ingredients of "real" community?[49] According to Wuthnow, "True community comes about when people play different roles and thus become interdependent" and when they are aware of needs outside the group: "Only by focusing explicit attention on the character of community and on the needs of the wider society are small groups likely to realize their potential for creating a genuine sense of community." It is unclear whether members of the small group I observed ever achieved this level of awareness, including how their needs might connect to the needs of the wider society.

Nevertheless, the journey of infertility[50] may not be the typical short-term and self-serving journey that Wuthnow describes. Rather, it seems to involve deep needs for membership and belonging. Beck invoked the sense of feeling "left out" of the "mundane and miraculous" process of having a baby. In some sense, people who resolve their infertility always feel a stronger sense of connection to their fellow sufferers than to fellow parents, for example. If RESOLVE provides a place to feel at home among similarly situated people, it may be more plausibly described as a club or haven than a community, at least according to Wuthnow's definition. However, I am not prepared to adopt this definition for the group of people I observed. I think other functions of RESOLVE meetings keep open the possibility of community.

Support Group or Public Discussion?

RESOLVE's monthly meetings are hard to categorize because they had different parts: the first part was more like a private support group and the second part was more of an informational public presentation and discussion. The small, living room discussion groups, which I was not permitted to attend as a researcher, lacked the public component. They were not open to just anyone who wanted to show up, and they did not, to my knowledge, have presentations by outside speakers. They were designated solely for the emotional support of their preregistered members. From my individual interviews, I also learned that the living room support groups tended to be more competitive and intrusive.[51]

One way to interpret RESOLVE's monthly meetings is as larger versions of the living room support groups, with the added distinctions of more fixed agendas, more directed conversations (by therapists/discussion leaders), and more fluid attendance, with group members more likely to remain strangers to each other. Yet in other ways, RESOLVE monthly meetings left space for something more. The public nature of the meetings provided at least the potential for spontaneous, broader concerns to be raised by whoever happened to be in attendance. The meetings provided opportunities for discussion with physicians and industry representatives, with at least the potential for critical questions to be raised. The meetings offered opportunities to discuss controversial topics, to see different aspects of the infertility industry, and to talk about larger societal issues.

On balance, however, most people came to the monthly meetings for emotional support, to share their stories, and to have their stories validated by others. In the words of RESOLVE's copresident, they were each other's "balcony people," cheering each other on and affirming each other and thereby providing a positive, uplifting presence in each other's lives through difficult times. "Basement people," in contrast, are the critics and naysayers who bring others down. The copresident concluded by saying RESOLVE had always been full of "balcony people" for her, and she hoped that others in the group would come to feel that way too. She explained that the idea of "balcony people" had come from a book by that title, although she never mentioned that it is an evangelical Christian inspirational book.[52]

Indeed, this understanding of the function of RESOLVE meetings as a place to receive affirmation and unconditional support closely echoes Wuthnow's description of self-help groups as "elevat[ing] the acceptance of individual opinion to a high art. . . . There can be no right or wrong interpretations. . . . The result is an exceptional level of tolerance for diversity, which of course is one reason why people are attracted to these groups. . . . Every view enjoys equal authority, no matter how unhelpful or unrealistic it may be."[53] While RESOLVE meetings were notably accepting and tolerant, there were some right and wrong interpretations of infertility (for example, it is an illness deserving of compassion rather than a psychological fabrication deserving of stigma), and some right and wrong positions on whether infertility treatments should be covered by insurance. In other words, substantive values operated at the meetings and in the larger organization. People were being educated into holding a particular set of definitions embodying a particular set of views.

Moreover, even though people did not use the forum of RESOLVE meetings to develop a critical perspective on any aspect of the infertility industry, they inevitably engaged in conversation with each other about issues larger than their individual desire to have a baby. People learned from each other, and the public nature of the monthly meetings helped to shape decision making. I am not prepared to label RESOLVE meetings a "subaltern counter public,"[54] using Nancy Fraser's often quoted terminology, although some elements of RESOLVE meetings probably fit her description. Foremost among these elements is the fact that meetings were a discursive space for the formulation of interests, such as how infertility should be defined apart from or in opposition to how society generally defines it. Given these subtle challenges to Wuthnow's model, it would be inaccurate to reduce the functions of RESOLVE's monthly meetings to those of merely a self-help group.

Many metaphors capture the functions of RESOLVE meetings: forum, club, community, public sphere, and so forth. Insofar as RESOLVE monthly meetings were public discussions, listening to these conversations as a participant/observer helped me to see connections between individuals' choices and larger social trends. As Nina Eliasoph suggests, listening to the interpersonal exchanges in public discussions—the "in between"—tells us more about how people engage with their society than investigating only subjective beliefs (the "inside") or social structures (the "outside").[55]

Did RESOLVE meetings serve as a site of critical conversation about ART and infertility? Would they satisfy Wuthnow's expectation that "people also need to hear tough, critical advice and to be called to follow high moral principles, rather than taking the course that simply makes them feel good"?[56] These questions, as well as the question of whether these are valid goals for RESOLVE, remain to be answered.

THREE

Public Discussions
of Infertility

Community Norms in
One Group's Quest

Individuals in Conversation:
Sharing, Finding, Creating Values

The People Who Attended

A core group of people attended the monthly RESOLVE meetings and symposia. Although some people came only once or twice, considerable continuity prevailed from month to month, and many returning members became friendly with each other, often staying after the meetings ended to talk informally in the greeting area outside the classrooms, where a table was always set up to display literature from RESOLVE and other sources, such as pharmaceutical companies, and to hold an array of food and drinks. I saw only one nonwhite attendee at any of the meetings, an African American woman who spoke during the peer discussion of her exhaustion at a very long struggle with infertility. She also expressed a loneliness, having worn out all her friends talking about her problem. She came to only a single meeting.

Most of the people who came to these evening meetings were professionals. Attendees identified themselves as teachers, nutritionists, managers, marketing directors, dental hygienists, social workers, ministers, and engineers, among other occupations. People often came directly from work to the meetings, wearing scrubs or suits and tailored skirts, carrying briefcases, and sipping smoothies purchased on the way. The majority of attendees were married couples. Virtually all of the others were women who came by themselves but spoke about not only their struggles but also those of their husbands.

In the comfortable, carpeted space provided by a suburban Atlanta hospital, members of this local RESOLVE chapter came together, got to know each other, and offered each other support and encouragement. During the peer group discussions, individuals—usually women—frequently solicited advice from each other and the discussion leader. For example, one woman and her husband reported deciding to seek a second opinion from a reproductive endocrinologist based on the specific advice and encouragement offered by several discussion group participants.[1] Group members had affirmed the woman's and her husband's suspicion that her regular ob-gyn physician, although claiming to specialize in infertility problems, might miss something crucial in her diagnosis and treatment that a specialist in reproductive endocrinology would catch. The discussion leader responded approvingly to the couple's decision, commending them for taking this next step and reiterating the benefits of RESOLVE meetings for encouraging people to seek out the help and resources they need.

At a later meeting, this woman, in turn, offered advice to another woman about the value of prayer in coping with infertility. The woman receiving the advice was a newcomer to the group and had just learned that her most recent cycle of in vitro fertilization (IVF) had failed, bringing her to an "all-time low" in her life.[2] She shook her head eagerly at the suggestion offered, admitting that she too used prayer, although no longer to ask for a child but to ask for the strength to endure the ordeal of infertility regardless of its outcome.

The Values of the Group

At RESOLVE meetings, members learned from each other how to interpret infertility, how to navigate the life crisis that it often precipitated, and how to emerge from it with an intact self and an intact marriage. The learning process was not hit or miss but received direction and structure from the more experienced RESOLVE leaders. These volunteers served as the link between the local chapter and the national office and thus most directly embodied or represented the organization's formal values. They followed national's lead in emphasizing the importance of insurance coverage, for example, but also drew on personal experiences with infertility and professional training (many were counselors of one kind or another) in giving guidance to other members. The leaders facilitated discussion and answered questions but did not by themselves determine the group's values.

In my individual interviews with RESOLVE members, I questioned people about their views of RESOLVE and about specific meetings. Individual members offered diverse assessments of these sessions: some people were pleasantly surprised by what they found at RESOLVE meetings, others were disappointed and even frustrated. However, participants rarely expressed negative opinions during meetings. Critical remarks emerged more openly in the individual interview setting. I also conducted a few interviews with individuals dealing with infertility who decided not to become RESOLVE members, and I asked them about their views of the group.

Individuals generally self-selected to join (or not to join) RESOLVE based on their prior understanding of its reputation. This is not to suggest that individuals who attended the monthly meetings always found what they were looking for or that all preconceptions about RESOLVE were confirmed. Whatever RESOLVE's real or perceived mission, the individuals who attended the monthly meetings were influenced by each other's presence and the discussions that occurred in that space. In the emotionally charged atmosphere of sharing problems and seeking solutions, people reflected on their personal values and tried to articulate what was important to them. Group sessions inevitably both drew out existing feelings and beliefs and provided people with new insights.

Several themes emerged from the discussions at the monthly meetings, the Saturday adoption symposium, and the interviews. The themes that seem best to represent how RESOLVE members defined what is significant in the experience of infertility include increased compassion for infertility and heightened awareness of others' problems, commiseration about the pain of unwanted moral judgments and a rejection of moralizing, a shared belief in the importance of self-education and empowerment, and an ambivalence about exhaustive efforts to achieve pregnancy. Indeed, one of the group's dynamic processes was the formulation and articulation of these group norms. Individuals who came to these meetings because they were in the midst of deliberating about decisions and dealing with problems looked to each other for cues about how to navigate these issues, including what resources to use, what priorities to adopt, how to interpret the experience, and how to orient themselves toward the outside world.

Discussion leaders' explicit advice undoubtedly influenced group members' ideas about how to move forward through infertility and how to handle other people, especially family and friends. The norms also emerged out of the particular constellation of individuals who attended the meetings during the year I did my research, their background beliefs, and their past experiences. A different group of people in a different time and place would have conducted a different conversation. Because this was an organic grouping of people embedded in their sociocultural contexts, RESOLVE meetings also gave voice to larger influences that shape many cultural norms about how to deal with infertility. However, the range of these norms was somewhat narrow, as the vast majority of attendees were white and middle or upper-middle class. The group did not lack diversity in priorities, interpretations, and opinions, but the group's values must be read in light of the particular social location of most of its members.[3]

Infertility Brings Greater Empathy and Inclusiveness

One woman came to a meeting in early January 2001 and shared some of the problems she was having with her in-laws, her mother-in-law in particular. She had come by herself. She was a well-dressed woman, probably in her mid-thirties, wearing wool slacks and diamond earrings. She spoke clearly and thoughtfully, telling a story about a family heirloom rocking chair. Her mother-in-law, owner of the rocking chair, had recently painted five little flowers on the chair's back and had explained that the flowers represented her five grandchildren: three existing grandchildren and two hoped-for grandchildren that she wanted this woman to have. The woman explained with exasperation, perhaps repeating an actual or imagined conversation with her mother-in-law, "We're doing the best we can! What more do you expect?"[4]

Infertility is seldom a problem that can be kept private. Before too long, family and friends inevitably ask, "So, when are you planning to have children?" And when doctors' visits, tests, shots, procedures, and/or adoption proceedings interfere with work schedules, coworkers and bosses eventually tend to find out. Even when the infertility problem did not become public, participants in the RESOLVE meetings widely reported feeling more vulnerable to comments and questions from others—for example, one woman used the metaphor of having a thin skin and falling apart at the slightest provocation —and that this vulnerability had produced some changes in their outlooks.

"I never want to forget that pain," said a discussion leader who had resolved her infertility through assisted reproductive technologies (ART).[5] She explained that going through infertility had made her much more aware of the insensitivity of certain comments and assumptions and that the memory of that experience made her sympathize with others currently going through it. Many participants in group discussion noted how much more conscious they had become of child-centered events, like the celebration of Mother's Day or Father's Day in churches, and wondered aloud at how child-centered events and child-centered conversations impacted the inevitable sufferers of infertility who often exist anonymously among their fertile peers. One woman related the memory of her minister asking all the mothers in the church to stand up and be recognized on Mother's Day and the resultant anguish she felt while staying seated.

Significantly, compassion was always extended to group members who were experiencing secondary infertility (having difficulty conceiving a second child) even though these couples often felt the need to ask group members' permission to be present. In response to one such a request, the discussion leader reiterated RESOLVE's commitment to support all types of infertility. She sympathetically described the "in-between state" that sufferers of secondary infertility experience, the difficulties of being "neither fully accepted by the infertile world nor fully understood by the fertile world."[6] Yet she reassured this man and woman that they would be welcome at RESOLVE.[7]

Thus, the emotional pain of the infertility experience seemed to increase individuals' capacity for empathy, at least for fellow sufferers of infertility. It heightened their awareness of and sensitivity to others' problems and encouraged a compassionate orientation regarding infertility of all kinds. Inclusiveness and respect for individuals' suffering were norms that clearly emerged in group interactions I observed.

Moralizing Is Unhelpful and Unwelcome

On numerous occasions, I heard people complain about the comment, "If God wants you to have a child, you will." Participants at monthly meetings were generally very conscious of the kinds of rationalizations, theological or not, that fertile people tend to apply to the infertility experience. Although insensitive comments often were deemed to be "well intentioned" and attributed to ignorance or not knowing what to say or how to help, group members at other times clearly disapproved of the moral tenor of other people's comments.

A regular attendee explained that she resented how people seemed so appreciative and approving of her decision to consider adoption but that the same people had been more skeptical about her pursuit of therapy through ART. She said that she was "not trying to save the world by considering adoption" but was "just trying to have a child." She also said that she believed some "stigma" was still attached to infertility treatments.[8]

An often-quoted RESOLVE pamphlet, *Managing Family and Friends*, which was always available on the literature table at monthly meetings, criticizes a hypothetical question from a friend or family member for its not-so-hidden judgment: "When are you going to stop concentrating on your career and start a family?" According to the pamphlet, this question is offensive because it "implies, of course, that your priorities are wrong or that you are selfish." It then offers two suggestions for an effective response that were referenced more than once during the discussions I attended: (1) "I don't believe that my job and a family are mutually exclusive. My career is advancing, and I'm very happy with my work. When we feel the time is right, we will consider starting our family"; and (2) "Right now I have two careers: one is my job, which you know about, and the other is trying to become pregnant. You probably wouldn't believe how exhausting and time-consuming infertility treatment can be; it really feels like a second job." Because the pamphlet is intended to educate RESOLVE members' friends and family, it also offers an alternative question that demonstrates greater sensitivity: "You used to talk about combining a career and a family. How are those plans coming along?"

While group members clearly interpreted certain comments from family and friends as containing an inappropriate moral judgment, sometimes the moral judgment in a question or comment was considered more ambiguous. For example, a couple experiencing secondary infertility expressed their disgust at some friends who used the "dreaded Christmas letter" to announce their third pregnancy, which was unplanned. The letter read, "I guess God decided to bless us again because we're such good parents." Because this woman and her husband were having trouble getting pregnant again, the woman saw the statement as having obvious implications: "Well, I guess that means we're not very good parents."[9] The lingering stigma of infertility may have influenced how such comments were interpreted, regardless of how they were intended. "Curse" is a plausible opposite of "blessing." Yet on this and similar occasions, other members of the group and the discussion leader offered a gentle challenge, reminding everyone that "life goes on" among those in the "fertile world": "You can't expect people not to talk about their kids or their unexpected pregnancies."[10]

These examples suggest that group members were very attuned to the moral judgments of others and viewed the RESOLVE meetings as a safe haven where they and their problems would not be judged. Group leaders explicitly and frequently assisted members in finding ways to protect themselves against unhelpful judgments by others and to deal with feelings of guilt and disappointment. Beyond that, moralizing about infertility or infertility treatments was clearly seen as inappropriate and unwelcome.

Empowerment through Self-Education and Emotional Awareness

Along with a sense of compassion for each other and for people struggling with infertility generally, another clear value that emerged in the discussions was the importance of self-education and empowerment. At a very basic level, the monthly meetings assumed that attendees were educated, motivated, and effective individuals—informed consumers, not passive patients. They had facility with the Internet, knowledge of the latest medical research, and a proactive stance toward treatment and toward the doctor-patient relationship. Physicians who addressed the group used scientific and technical language, presented graphs of outcomes from research studies, showed slides of complicated surgical procedures, and discussed the latest protocols, all with seemingly little translation for a lay audience.[11] This generally high level of scientific literacy, active orientation toward treatment, and appreciation for technological advances in medicine constituted some of the more obvious places where socioeconomic status likely influenced the group's norms.

When I asked one of the copresidents of RESOLVE of Georgia in an interview which of the year's meetings she thought had been the most effective, she responded that one of them would have to be the October 2000 "Ask the Experts" meeting: "So many couples really want that information. Plus, you've got six physicians from five different clinics, presenting different views. [At] the Q&A session . . . there were *thirty* questions that were answered! It was like a free consultation. . . . But it's wonderful to see that one of them does not have *the* answer. There are a lot of different views, a lot of different protocols."[12] Left unsaid was how a person might navigate among all these different views and protocols. But self-education seemed to hold the key. Knowing more is better. One speaker recommended keeping files labeled by topic (for example, medical, psychological, ethical, moral, and religious) for information obtained from the Internet.[13]

Another physician with a Web site and weekly chat room about infertility lectured on the "metanalysis" of medical studies and "evidence-based medicine."[14] His stated goal was to give the audience the knowledge and tools they needed to assess which treatments would work best for them and more generally to "partner" with their doctors in the decision-making process. Although he touted the benefits of evidenced-based medicine, he also noted that "lack of evidence does not equal lack of effectiveness." Thus, in clinical decision making, he recommended asking, "What is my risk? What is my chance of responding? What is the treatment's feasibility in my MD's practice? What are my values?" In response to the last question, he said, "I can't make these decisions for you. This is such personal stuff. I can only educate you about the choices."[15]

In addition to providing the space in which members can become educated about the options for medical treatment, RESOLVE meetings also provided explicit instruction on how to deal with feelings, how to protect oneself emotionally, and how to maintain a healthy and happy relationship with one's spouse or partner. Therapists addressed the group more often than physicians did during the year I attended and were usually more explicitly directive in their advice. The therapists' wisdom was often adopted as the group's wisdom, reiterated among members and organizational leaders in subsequent group discussions. For example, discussion participants were told to identify their feelings and accept them as normal, that it is okay to feel jealous, angry, hateful, helpless, frustrated, and so on. Therapists also liked to give participants "absolution" from attending all baby showers and child-centered events, telling people to "ignore what convention seems to require" and protect the self, which is "grieving and vulnerable."[16]

Members seemed to want to know this information, often asking directly for advice. In response to a question about how to handle insensitive comments, one discussion leader/therapist recommended that people divide hurtful comments into three categories. (1) There are the "unthinking" comments of people "who don't really know you that well and who don't intend to hurt your feelings." For these comments, largely made out of ignorance, she recommended a very brief reply, such as "Thanks for your concern." (2) Then there are the comments from people "who are really close to you, who are trying to help, but just say the wrong thing." For these people, she recommended putting in the effort to educate them about infertility and to "be clear about your expectations and boundaries." Tell close friends and well-meaning family members what specifically would be the most helpful. (3) Finally, there are those people who are indeed mean-spirited in what they say and shamelessly exploit the infertility experience for an invidious comparison. For these persons, she recommended a "gloves-off" approach. She said to confront the person outright and "say that what you're going through is really painful and that you don't want to compete with them about it . . . then watch them backpedal all the way to New York, because no one wants to be perceived as insensitive."[17]

Finally, one important aspect of empowering individuals who attended RESOLVE meetings was encouraging couples to work through infertility decisions together, as couples. The therapists/discussion leaders reasoned that individuals differ in what they need but that greater awareness of these differences can help foster closeness and support. The group accepted this logic and embraced the ideals of egalitarian decision making and mutual respect within a marriage/partnership. The group also embraced the vision of the couple as a self-protecting island, standing together against outside judgments.

Most basically, the group clearly accepted the idea that knowledge is power, and the more knowledge one can gather about the options for treating infertility, the better. Similarly, the more aware one can be of one's emotional state, the more prepared one can be to deal with the insensitivity of others from a position of strength.

If there was general agreement about the value of knowing more and educating oneself about various emotional issues, there seemed to be less agreement about how many treatments, how long to try, or how much money to spend. All matters of limit setting and decision making were addressed as areas of personal choice. The norm that seemed to govern these conversations was an unconditional acceptance for whatever an individual (couple) needed to do to "move forward" in the process of resolving infertility.

In explaining their decision to use ART, many people expressed the need to give it their "best try"[18] or to try "everything that medical science has to offer"[19] so they could live with themselves without any regrets. Others could not tolerate years of medical treatment or an indefinite number of medical interventions but still felt compelled to try something: "We both felt that we wanted to at least make an attempt so that if we looked back later, we could say we at least tried one time."[20] The avoidance of regret seemed to be an important motivator in decisions to use ART.

Some physicians seemed to exploit this desire or motivation, while others were more scrupulous about limiting medical interventions that they believed were not in the patient's best interest. For example, one physician who advertised his Web site and infertility chat room when he spoke at a monthly meeting held an online question-and-answer session (which I observed) shortly after his visit to RESOLVE. When someone asked how many intrauterine inseminations she should try in her efforts to get pregnant, his brief answer was, "As many as your budget will allow."[21] In contrast, the physicians who came for the October 2000 "Ask the Experts" meeting were very careful in answering questions. When asked why some fertility clinics do not accept women over age forty-two, the physicians responded straightforwardly about different clinics' "philosophies" with regard to using treatments that had a very low probability of success. They also reassured the group, with considerable sensitivity and compassion, that the refusal to see older patients was motivated not by a desire to protect a clinic's success statistics (because age groups are always separated out for national reporting) but by a desire to provide good patient care.[22]

Participants at RESOLVE meetings questioned to some degree the idea that exhaustive effort is always good, although the clearest voices contesting this norm often seemed to come from people finished with or near the end of their journey with ART. At the February 2001 adoption symposium, for example, one couple admitted that they were now considering adoption after fifteen years of infertility treatments. After some in the audience gasped audibly, the couple explained with more fatigue than anger, "The doctors were always coming up with one more thing to try."[23] The discussion leader responded by saying that infertility treatments can be "seductive" and that she had felt liberated when she and her husband finally decided to stop trying to get pregnant and adopt. A therapist at an earlier monthly meeting also expressed a willingness to challenge the wisdom of exhaustive efforts and encouraged her audience to retake control of the decision-making process. She said infertility treatments were not about "keeping up with the Joneses. . . . You don't have to follow the doctor's plan or what somebody else is doing."[24]

In an interview, one RESOLVE member, now an adoptive mother, said, "I feel like screaming at people who go through all this medical [ART] stuff: 'Are you nuts? Do you know how satisfying [adoption] can be? Do you know that there are kids out there that need homes? Why are you all waiting for some perfect little thing?' It seems—the medical stuff seems so nuts to me right now."[25] Although she admitted that she was still in the "honeymoon period" with her child, she seemed sufficiently unhappy with her experience with ART to offer some generalizations. Criticizing some of the practices of the infertility industry, she later added, "I do feel like it's really become a field of moneymaking. . . . Most of the couples I've come across seem to be so emotionally tied up in it that they will go with whatever hope is given to them by the specialists that they are seeing."[26]

Another RESOLVE member, now also an adoptive mother, was much more tentative in her comments about the infertility industry generally but described her personal experience with medical treatments as a source of great disappointment: ART "made me feel like if I tried hard enough and had enough money, I would get pregnant, which didn't end up being true."[27]

Broader Themes

The public discussions I observed and interviews I conducted also featured other, less explicit themes. Broader ideas about gender, race, class, and consumerism constituted a less obvious part of the conversation than, for example, the painful isolation of infertility, but they provide useful lenses with which to view discussions about efforts to achieve pregnancy. Using these categories helps to illuminate how social contexts constrain, shape, and give meaning to individual choices and provides further insight into the values and commitments of this particular group. Similarly, religion and ethics formed a part of the conversation in important and subtle ways, although the discussions of religious questions—those involving both institutional religion and individual expressions of religious belief or spirituality—were at times surprisingly explicit. By ethics, I mean an identifiably normative inquiry into the rightness or wrongness of private choices and social practices. Again, listening to discussions of these topics provides insight into the values and commitments of the group and the role that RESOLVE played for its members.

Gender Differences

Participants in RESOLVE's monthly discussion meetings, which always included both women and men, often talked about how the experience of infertility is "different for women." Men, it was frequently said with humor, are "about a trimester behind" their wives in coming to the decision to seek a diagnosis for infertility, to seek treatment for infertility, to move from low-tech to high-tech treatment, and to begin considering adoption or a child-free life. Women are also more likely to research the treatment options "obsessively," according to the experiences reported at RESOLVE meetings, and to be more eager to get back on the "treadmill of infertility" after any treatment that does not result in a pregnancy.[28] In fact, trying several cycles of IVF back to back was not uncommon. Women, it would seem, are differently invested than men in becoming parents.[29]

This observation directly contradicts the conclusion of a study of RESOLVE members conducted by Judith Lasker and Susan Borg and reported in *In Search of Parenthood* (1987).[30] Lasker and Borg claim that men are more invested in using reproductive technologies than women and that women often acquiesce to their husbands' decision making. I encountered the opposite phenomenon, however: women were far more motivated and determined to try ART than were their husbands.

This higher level of motivation may have been related to women's different coping strategies for dealing with infertility generally. Speakers at meetings commonly assumed that women cope differently with infertility than do men. This difference usually was characterized by women's greater emotional awareness. "Women give voice to their feelings," explained a discussion leader/therapist. "Men tend to fear losing control."[31] Women are also believed to have trouble finding socially acceptable ways to vent their anger at infertility, while men typically try to "fix" their partner's disappointment rather than simply being present to offer support.[32] Different ways of coping can strain a relationship, but group members often talked about ways to keep the lines of communication open and to move forward together as a couple.[33]

Other perceived gender differences thought to explain women's greater motivation to try ART centered on women's and men's disparate sources of self-esteem and social worth. I conducted individual interviews with two discussion leaders who were also therapists. Each provided an especially blunt assessment of perceived gender differences along these lines. The female therapist explained, "I just think that [women] tend to get more into [ART] because I think we're more emotionally attuned, and I think . . . traditionally, men have worked and that's their production, and women have children, and that's their production and job in life. So as long as [a man is] working and making money and providing enough money to do the treatment stuff, then [his wife] can do everything. It's not so cut-and-dry, but as I look at all the reasons possibly why, I think men get their worth from work, and women typically get it from their relationships with people and their connections, and one of them is children."[34] Similarly, according to the male therapist, men are "so connected to our career and our work [but] typically a woman's sense of herself is related to relationships, children and parenting, the spouse. I think that's just part of . . . why it's so difficult for men to get on board" with treatment. He also said, "I think it's a God-given part of being a woman. . . . There's nothing more feminine than giving birth to a child."[35] Such stereotypical characterizations of "feminine" and "masculine" did not find their way into these therapists' public comments during RESOLVE meetings, however.

For their part, RESOLVE members often talked about the fact that diagnostic procedures and treatments for infertility are generally much more invasive for women than for men: "The reality is that gender roles are imbalanced when trying to achieve pregnancy."[36] As one woman said in an interview, "I still think it's completely invading and completely—I mean, you literally spread your legs in every aspect of your life—financially, emotionally, physically. You're just completely vulnerable to the world, and that's still the woman's part."[37] She also noted that public pity still goes to the woman who cannot get pregnant rather than to the couple that cannot have a child: "Everybody talked about 'Poor Sally Smith. She can't get pregnant.' It was never, 'Oh, poor Hal and Sally Smith.'" Moreover, she felt that when ART works, it "makes it good for women because you don't have that hole that you failed . . . or that you haven't succeeded."[38]

Not being able to "achieve" a pregnancy was very often compared to a sense of being excluded: as one participant put it at a meeting, "It's like a big club, and you can't get in that club."[39] That feeling of exclusion can strain female friendships in particular. One woman was very angry at a friend for complaining about an unplanned pregnancy and identified this anger as emanating from the fact that "I wasn't part of a club that I wanted to be a part of so badly."[40]

A *RESOLVE of Georgia Newsletter* article written by a man explicitly summarizes some of the implicit assumptions I found operating in group discussions: "Women are taught to expect to grow up and have a job called mommy. . . . For a man to truly understand a woman's feelings about infertility, he must, I believe, come to envision her feeling in terms of equivalent loss to himself. Imagine what it would be like to be unable to earn or even think about earning and producing what you would like. Imagine what your family and friends expect of you and what they would think."[41] Many of the women I interviewed expressed great disappointment at not being able to experience pregnancy. Their comments confirmed a lingering sense that women derive a significant sense of worth from their roles as mothers, regardless of other roles they fill or their success in their careers/employment. However, one woman I interviewed who is not a RESOLVE member talked at length about how she has come to see her "vocation" as not needing to include being a mother. She was proud to be an aunt and a godparent and was fulfilled in her work, which included teaching, something she described as a nurturing role.[42]

Women also seemed to see themselves as differently responsible for infertility, especially because of the sensitive issue of age. At the January 2001 meeting, a woman asked the discussion leader why she thought the incidence of infertility had increased in recent years. The discussion leader responded simply that women now tend to wait to "have babies" and "do career first."[43] In an interview, this leader elaborated her ideas about the causes of infertility: "Of course, one of the major factors is age—that we all, at this point, in this generation, tend to do career, get married later, wait later, and we know that a woman's reproductive health, . . . the quality of her eggs decreases as she ages. Maybe in years and years to come, women may try to get pregnant earlier."[44] The physicians who spoke at monthly meetings generally confirmed members' concerns about age. When asked how doctors know whether IVF is going to work, one physician replied definitively, "The strongest predictor is age." He also bluntly advised the women in the group, "If you're over thirty-eight, the most cost-effective plan is to use donor eggs."[45]

Women sometimes seemed defensive about the decision to delay childbearing or marriage, as if they owed someone an explanation for waiting. Introducing herself and her fiancé to the group, one woman explained that they had come to the meeting because they wanted to get a "jump start" on infertility issues because they were a "little older" and a "little late" in getting married.[46] Another woman was very upset that her doctor had "pretty much told me I waited too long" to try to conceive a child.[47] She was also upset that her mother and sisters bore children "later in life," which she defined as mid- to late thirties. She had always thought she would meet with the same results, so she had never thought about trying to have children until recently. She also described her frustration with coworkers who made assumptions about her childlessness: they assumed she did not like children or was "one of those people" who did not value family over career.

A final issue relevant to gender and gender differences was the issue of competition among women. Group members often relayed painful stories about feeling jealous of a sister, sister-in-law, friend, coworker, and/or subordinate employee who easily became pregnant. These women wondered why others had an easier time becoming pregnant and were mortified by feelings of jealousy and resentment. Some women made comparisons across generations, reflecting on how their mothers or mothers-in-law approached childbearing decisions and timing. In these latter cases, the women at times seemed to be reflecting on paths not taken, as if the choices available to women still amounted to either motherhood or career but not both.

I will return later in this chapter to the issue of competition among women and the idea of different paths. Participants at RESOLVE meetings never seriously questioned what women expected of themselves in terms of becoming mothers/fulfilling the role of mother. Discussion leaders/therapists and their beliefs about why women tend to pursue ART more aggressively than men generally reinforced stereotypical gender roles. RESOLVE members also did not tend to question the trend of delayed childbearing as anything more significant than a matter of personal choice and failed to explore the possibility, however remote, that societal structures be changed to enable women more easily to combine the aspirations of motherhood and career.

Socioeconomic Class

Only once during any of the monthly meetings or individual interviews did I hear class explicitly mentioned: a speaker at the adoption symposium, now an adoptive parent, recounted that she and her husband had "cleaned out" both sides of their family to finance seven years of infertility treatment: "And they were just working-class, middle-class people!"[48]

Nevertheless, class-specific expectations and assumptions were expressed at monthly meetings, often by discussion leaders, who cited long-term interaction with RESOLVE members or with people experiencing infertility generally as their basis of knowledge. For example, a physician addressing the group said, "The best patient is an educated patient, but luckily so many infertility patients are so well educated to begin with."[49] A therapist made a similar statement: "Probably many of you are involved in careers" and thus are "quite competent at coping with problems," but infertility requires a "new bag of tricks."[50] A physician who advertised his book and Web site repeatedly at the meeting seemed to flatter and encourage the group with his assessment that "people involved in RESOLVE not only resolve their infertility but they're more successful in getting what they want generally."[51]

In an interview, one therapist speculated about particular frustrations that accompany class-specific expectations, although he did not use the language of class: "A lot of these couples, I'm sure you've seen some of them, met some of them, they're very successful, educated, go-getters, and you take a couple like that that has succeeded in everything they've ever undertaken, and their body is not working the way God has created it to work. It really—the anxiety level" is high.[52] A therapist at the adoption symposium described himself and his wife as "DINKs" (dual income, no kids) who tried every available ART treatment before adopting two boys. As he spoke, he seemed to imply that his experience was not unique, but he may have had many points in common with his audience.[53]

Another indicator of the socioeconomic status of many RESOLVE members was simply the fact that for most, ART was an option. Despite the cost of infertility treatments, which can be several thousand dollars each and are usually paid out of pocket, most people who came to RESOLVE meetings seemed to possess the ability to obtain such treatments. One woman worried that "all this money was going towards treatments that did not work" but added, "Money is replaceable."[54] Financial limitations would not, it seemed, determine how many more cycles of IVF this couple attempted.[55] Numerous comments in the course of discussions and interviews also gave me a sense of what was affordable and/or within the realm of the possible for many people. For example, one woman mused that perhaps having a child "is not to be" and that their struggles with infertility are a "sign" that "maybe we're supposed to move to the Caribbean and hang out and enjoy life down there."[56]

Financial limits were more commonly discussed in the context of adoption, perhaps because that option tended to be considered only after an expensive course of infertility treatment had been pursued. Financial limitations surely affect many people's decisions about whether to pursue either ART or adoption, but the ordering of these priorities (first ART, then adoption or child-free living) seemed a very common background assumption. As one person stated at the adoption symposium, "Most people come to adoption after having spent a lot of money on infertility treatment, but there are many ways to finance an adoption."[57] During an interview, a woman in the process of undergoing treatment for infertility and considering using donor eggs stated, "Our doctors' advice to us along the way, which I think has been really valuable, is,

'Don't even start thinking down a path until you're there.' You just focus on what you need to do in the meantime."[58] She did not question his logic of trying (and finishing) treatment before moving on to adoption.

Despite the financial resources apparently available to many of the attendees at RESOLVE meetings, the cost of ART seemed to cause a great deal of resentment among users. Participants expressed frustration at having to pay so much for what others can have for free. A discussion leader who had success through ART expressed anger at having to spend money on ART when friends were buying new houses and cars.[59] This comparison was significant because members often talked about ART as a big-ticket consumer item—on the same order of magnitude as a vacation, for example. One woman without insurance coverage for her treatment lamented the financial trade-offs she and her husband had to make to pay for IVF: "This couple in our group therapy, they have everything covered. They go on vacations, and we think, 'Can you imagine how much better we'd be able to get with this if we just spent a week in the Cayman Islands?' But we can't do that."[60]

That people are willing to spend so much of their money to have a child speaks to the seriousness of their desire and suggests their willingness to make significant financial sacrifices—sacrifices that they see other members of the same socioeconomic class not having to make, and sacrifices that prioritize having children over highly prized material goods such as cars, houses, and vacations. However, the narrow range of people who can afford expensive infertility treatments out of pocket is also significant, as is the way they con-ceptualize ART as a consumer good. These observations may help to explain why people who try ART tend to try a lot of it. In other words, exhaustive efforts to achieve pregnancy may not be purely the function of the strength of someone's desire to have a child; they may also be at least partially a function of having the means to pursue a highly coveted consumer good and the fact that ART is often presented by specialists as an effective, rational, empower-ing, even self-actualizing use of technology—an image/rationale that appeals largely to middle- and upper-middle-class clientele.

As will be discussed at greater length in chapter 4, a "fit" arguably exists between the individuals who choose to use ART and the industry that pursues their business. The people who can afford to use ART typically think of themselves as having the ability to get what they want with enough effort or money. They tend to conceptualize infertility as an unjust thwarting of the expectation that hard work leads to desired results. At the same time, the infertility industry has positioned itself to fulfill these expectations, to rectify the wrong done by infertility, and to satisfy the need to be "doing something" to repair the self-conceptions of ordinarily successful and effective individuals.

The infertility industry clearly is a highly competitive market, actively pursuing clients who can pay for its high-end services and more thoroughly driven by profit than by the idea of alleviating the medical problems of the diverse population of people who suffer from infertility.[61] There is little sense that the arrival of ART is a public good, on a par with a new vaccine or basic prenatal care, for example—something that will benefit the population generally.

Indeed, rarely if ever did participants in the monthly meetings articulate an awareness of how infertility might affect people who cannot afford to pay for treatment. Insofar as infertility and access to ART were ever viewed as problems of social justice, the discussion leaders at RESOLVE meetings were the most likely to frame the need for insurance coverage in terms of how it would benefit everyone.

Consumerism

Just as members seldom used the language of class in their discussions, neither did they talk about how consumerism might be a part of their experience. Being an "informed consumer" was a natural, unquestioned background assumption of most RESOLVE members. While no one wanted doctors or fertility clinics to take advantage of them, few people considered the larger picture—how their individual choices to pursue ART might be influenced by the booming infertility industry that has sprung up to meet their needs. The phenomenon of consumerism was not an issue that rose to the level of the group's explicit consideration.

However, one evening's presentation (on navigating the Internet for resources about infertility) seemed particularly relevant to considering the impact of consumerism on pursuing infertility treatment. The night's two main speakers had substantially different attitudes toward the Internet. The first speaker advised the group to be very cautious about privacy, offering a lengthy warning about cookies, which are "sneaky peeks into your computer" that show where on the Internet a person has visited, how long he or she has stayed, and so forth—information that can be shared or sold. He told the group to be aware of what Web sites were trying to sell them. He also talked about how information on the Internet is totally unregulated and gave a general caution about the different interests of "objective versus subjective sources." Without naming them as either objective or subjective, he listed as examples of information sources pharmaceutical companies, private practices, state colleges and universities, private/religious colleges and universities, hospitals and clinics, foundations, nonprofit organizations, and state and federal government agencies.[62]

By contrast, the second speaker was very enthusiastic about the Internet, including advertising specifically tailored to an individual's past visits and purchases. He agreed with the first speaker that the information on the Internet is unregulated but offered some tips on how to tell good information from "garbage." For example, he provided the names and Web addresses of online sources that physicians use (e.g., Medline and Grateful Med, as well as his informational Web site, IVF.com) and then noted that "dot-edus are not your best source of information [about infertility]. Universities are not the cutting edge. They're about ten years behind."[63] Instead, he steered the group to the dot-coms as a better source of information.

Since he had encouraged group members to visit his Web site, I did so shortly after the meeting on the assumption that some other audience members would do the same. His Web site contained a link to a bookstore that sold products related to infertility treatment. The text under the bookstore icon read, "Crass consumerism has invaded our website. For those who like to shop, we have a few items you may wish to consider."[64]

During the presentation itself, no one seemed particularly critical of the second speaker. In fact, one couple stated to the group that they had come to the meeting for the express purpose of hearing this physician speak, as they knew of him by reputation. In addition, no one in any of my individual interviews raised concerns about that meeting, although I did not have a chance to speak individually to every person in attendance. Only in the interview with one of the copresidents did an issue emerge—an acknowledgment that the second speaker had been dismissive of the concerns of a woman who was worried about using Clomid, a fertility drug that regulates ovulation, because some studies had linked the drug to birth defects. The physician responded to her concerns by saying, among other things, "You hear infertility drugs cause cancer. They don't, they don't," a response that the copresident described as "sort of pooh-pooh[ing]" the question.[65]

In striking contrast to the relative silence during RESOLVE meetings about the pressure to consume ART, one woman I interviewed, not a RESOLVE member, was quite willing to make general critical comments on this point. She explained her decision not to join RESOLVE by saying that she perceived the women in the group as "all desperate to conceive." She discussed her brief experience with infertility treatment, including its impact on her husband, and explained that her worries about not being able to have a baby had combined with the overeager attitude of her infertility doctor to create what she called "hysteria": "It was one of those bad hand-in-glove combinations, and I just bought it."[66] She said her doctor was very "goal-oriented" and would not entertain any discussion outside the goal of conception: his attitude seemed to her to say, "You're here to have a baby, right? You're either going to do it this way or no way." This woman's husband reacted very negatively to their doctor's approach, and she eventually came to share his impression and to feel "pressured."

In another interview, a RESOLVE member and former leader who remarked that she had to be careful about what she said "because I do to a certain degree represent RESOLVE" commented regarding the consumption of ART, "I think there's a lot of money that's being wasted out there that if people—couples—were better educated and were able to push some of the emotions aside would question more some of the recommendations that are being made."[67]

While these women articulated a more critical perspective of the infertility industry based on experience, most RESOLVE participants were not willing to generalize in this way. Intense anger was often expressed at individual physicians for the way they handled—or mishandled—their infertility patients' care,[68] but few people seemed willing or able to reflect on the interaction of their needs with a for-profit medical establishment or with the wider influences of a consumerist culture. Nor did RESOLVE meetings seem to encourage this type of reflection.

The Absent Issue of Race

"I wanted a white baby like everybody else," explained one adoptive mother forthrightly in an interview.[69] She obtained a white infant through domestic adoption. As with class and consumerism, the issue of race only rarely arose explicitly during group discussions or formal presentations. However, in some ways, the priority of having a child of the same race was always a background assumption of the conversation. In the vast majority of discussions I observed, this assumption meant white.

At the February 2001 adoption symposium, which was held in a large downtown Atlanta church and attracted well over a hundred attendees, there was only one nonwhite person in the room—an African American woman who ran an adoption agency, Roots, specializing in special-needs adoptions of African American children. She led a session on special-needs adoption, which was the most poorly attended of the symposium's presentations. No potential adoptive parents came to the session, only other agency workers and organizational leaders—a total of five people. The agency director explained that "special needs" is a federal definition that includes any African American male child older than one, any African American female child older than five, and sibling groups. "Special needs" also includes children in the foster care system and children with health problems or disabilities.

It was not clear to me that the symposium attendees as a whole knew of the definition of "special needs" or, if they did, why interest in the session was so low. The obvious explanation was that it competed with sessions on domestic and international adoption procedures that attracted dozens of people each. I had assumed that "special needs" meant exclusively physical or mental disabilities. It would seem that "special needs" is really code for "undesirable" or "hard to place."

In addition to the formal presentations at the symposium, which included a nuts-and-bolts orientation regarding adoption; separate interactive sessions on domestic, international, and special-needs adoptions; transitioning from infertility treatment to adoption; parenting adopted children; and "Telling Your Child's Adoption Story: What, When, and How to Tell," attendees had access to a great deal of written literature, including numerous fliers and magazines set out on tables.[70] Some of this literature more plainly addressed the issue of race than did any of the speakers. For example, one of the fliers, produced by Adoption Information Services of Lawrenceville, Georgia, bore the title *How to Play the Adoption Game Financially and Emotionally* and began, "Remember you are not buying a baby. You are paying for services to get a child here." The text went on to explain the fee structure: "Amount depends on the race and age of the child, typically $2,500 to $10,000 for African-American or biracial; $10,000 to $30,000 for Caucasian, Hispanic, or Asian." That the fees ranged according to race, however, certainly hinted that one was buying a baby and that some babies were worth more than others.

A frank discussion of how race may be a factor in the demand for ART versus the demand for adoption did not occur in any of the sessions I attended at the adoption symposium, nor did I ever observe such a discussion at any of the regular monthly RESOLVE meetings. That parents desired children of the same race struck me as the kind of assumption that people did not believe required interrogation and that even mentioning it might have been in poor taste. The pervasiveness of this assumption at least partially explains the ordering of so many people's priorities in dealing with infertility: first try treatment using one's own sperm and eggs. If that does not succeed, the next step might be to consider using a sperm or egg donor matched for race and other physical traits. If using a sperm or egg donor is impossible or not compatible with the couple's values, the next step might be to consider adopting a white U.S. infant or, if that proves too difficult, adopting from a nation that can supply a white infant (for example, an Eastern European country). Of course, people adopt all the time from Asia, South America, and other places that can supply nonwhite infants. Had there been the interest, the adoption symposium could have framed a session around respecting the cultural heritages of adopted children, which might have provided an opportunity to question the assumption that adopted children should ideally be the same race as their parents.

Instead of a broader discussion about race, however, I observed some frank comments about how both ART and adoption are properly and logically understood as meeting personal needs, not serving social justice.[71] As one discussion participant stated, "I'm not trying to save the world by considering adoption. . . . I'm just trying to have a child."[72] People were, in fact, explicitly discouraged during the special-needs adoption session from approaching the adoption process with a "hero mentality"—that is, with the intention of "rescuing" unwanted children, both for the parents' sake and for the well-being of their future children. One adoptive mother explained that it was psychologically unhealthy to pursue adoption for these reasons, however noble doing so may seem in the abstract. These remarks resonate strongly with the arguments of feminist ethicist and theologian Christine Gudorf, who suggests that it is disingenuous to portray adoption as saintly self-sacrifice and to underestimate the strong and natural motive to have a child of one's own.[73] The people I observed also expressed a pervasive sense that it may be unfair as well as unrealistic to expect an already disadvantaged population (those experiencing infertility) to shoulder a disproportionate burden of the world's children who need homes.

The belief that the infertile are an already disadvantaged population that should not be called on to adopt the world's "unwanted" children, while somewhat convincing on the surface, requires greater scrutiny than it ever received in my observation. For example, what does it suggest about society's views of children? Or, more precisely, what does it suggest about white, middle- and upper-middle-class secularized views of children? Rather than being viewed as "gifts" to which we are owed no particular entitlement, children are more like possessions or commodities whose price is set by the laws of supply and demand. Though this may be a coarser formulation than any attendee at the adoption symposium would have been comfortable articulating, I believe it is the only thing that plausibly explains why some children are more "adoptable" and affordable than others.

In addition, what does the belief that the "unfairness" of infertility should not be compounded by the unfairness of adopting the world's unwanted children suggest about this group's views of social justice? Has justice been reduced to simply getting what we want for ourselves rather than providing to members of society what is their due, such as the nurturing care of a family for every child? Whether this limited conception of justice is a white, middle- or upper-middle-class, secularized view or a more pervasively American attitude is impossible to judge with certainty. But these kinds of questions were generally absent from the conversation at RESOLVE meetings.

Religion

Religion was mentioned with some regularity during the monthly meetings, often in the context of participants expressing disappointment or frustration that their religion disapproved of a certain form of ART. Insofar as religious institutions and religious leaders render moral judgments about certain paths for resolving infertility, they were regarded as unhelpful. During the year prior to my research, RESOLVE had conducted a symposium on "Faith Issues and Infertility." As a pastoral counselor related during an interview, a Catholic priest led one of the sessions at the symposium, and "I don't know if it was related to his personality, but there were a lot of couples that left the group that were pretty angry and hurt. . . . I think he was pretty much against any kind of reproductive intervention. . . . They were really offended by what he said, and that's my experience for a lot of couples, and what I found . . . is that many churches are really not helpful for these couples."[74] Moreover, the counselor said, many religions do not understand or accept what people are doing, which can underscore their sense of isolation and guilt.[75]

During an interview, one of the RESOLVE copresidents discussed religion's role in decisions about ART: "Very often, your faith does not believe that the option you're considering is right, is biblical. And then you struggle with, 'Well, if I go through with this, then what?' " She elaborated, "I was just reading an article about religion, and how [for] different religions, certain types of reproductive technologies are considered okay, some are not. So, you know, if you're a person of faith, that clouds your decision and really makes an inner conflict. . . . People that have never experienced it or don't have the knowledge of it don't know what an emotional, traumatic crisis it can be, trying to sift through all these decisions to finally have a child. And I just feel like we are a blessed society to be able to have these options to build a family."[76] Other RESOLVE members echoed this appreciation for "options." As one woman stated, "I hear there's a lot of people who think [ART is] wrong and have problems with it, and I just think, you know, if you were in my shoes, you would change your tune real fast. . . . I can't imagine anyone who ended up in this situation wouldn't be glad that there are options there for them."[77]

Group members generally seemed to perceive religious organizations and leaders as failing to appreciate the benefits of options for building families. Religious officials were seen as too willing to judge the use of reproductive technologies, usually without firsthand knowledge of the experience of infertility. In response to the accusation that people who use ART are "playing God," discussion participants would reply, "If God gave us the technology, then why not use it?"[78]

In addition, churches were perceived primarily as family-oriented places that alienated people experiencing infertility. On more than one occasion, discussion participants shared stories about avoiding church altogether or particular church services that attracted a lot of children. A Protestant minister and his wife came to only one RESOLVE meeting, on the topic of "Coping with the Holidays," and explained that for them, the Christmas holiday was also the anniversary of the removal of an ectopic pregnancy.[79] The husband spoke movingly about the particular challenges of his professional role; about how Christmas is supposed to be a time of hopeful expectancy, as the center of it is a pregnant mother waiting for the arrival of her baby; and how at odds he felt personally with the meaning of this holiday and its happy spirit.[80]

A woman undergoing treatment for infertility stated in an interview, "I wish that churches would have more of a ministry [for the infertile], and yet churches are so focused on children."[81] She also pointed out that RESOLVE could not offer the kind of religiously based support she sought because it had to appeal to "the masses."

Despite the common disappointment in organized religion for its unhelpful moral judgments and/or lack of meaningful support for people experiencing infertility, participants in RESOLVE meetings were still interested in a typical preoccupation of religion: explaining why bad things happen to good people. These so-called theodicy questions (Why do the good suffer and the wicked prosper? What kind of God allows the good to suffer?) were a remarkably frequent topic of the group's conversations and seemed to be motivated by anger at suffering perceived as undeserved. As often as not, discussion participants expressed a generalized anger at the injustice of infertility rather than a specific anger at God. For example, one husband who attended the meetings regularly with his wife explained that what really made him angry was "watching TV and seeing a story about a sixteen-year-old with her second child who doesn't know who the father is. It's not fair!"[82] Another husband responded, "Being angry at injustice is a good thing. It's *not* fair. The world has things in it that aren't fair or just."[83]

However, many discussion participants framed their anger at infertility in explicitly theological terms, including one woman who speculated, "People say that God gives us children, but there's a big hole between" people with children and the infertile. She relayed a news story she had heard about some abused foster children, one of whom was a four-year-old whose teeth had rotted out, and conveyed her frustration with the fact that people who would be caring parents cannot conceive children: "I can't make it work! I can't reconcile it."[84] Another woman described the spiritual questioning prompted by her experience with a miscarriage after she had beaten the odds by getting pregnant through IVF: "I guess for me it was just too much of a tease to go through the stress of 'Oh, my gosh! We only have a 6–8 percent chance and then I get pregnant and lose it!' was just really distressing. I had a period of probably a good two months where I was definitely clinically depressed. But it was kind of a—oh, I don't know how I would term it, a sort of cleansing time for me, too, because I can remember laying in my bed, looking out the window at the same tree constantly thinking about why did this happen. Why did God let this happen? Why couldn't I just not have gotten pregnant and the IVF just didn't work?"[85] This woman did not abandon her religion as a result of her experience. After a successful adoption, she articulated the ways her faith had been renewed and even strengthened.

Many people who attended RESOLVE meetings found religion a complicated topic. Religious or spiritual questioning seemed a common outgrowth of the experience of infertility,[86] but participants by no means expressed a monolithic view of religion as either a negative or positive influence. When religion could be a source of support or strength or insight, it was mentioned favorably. For example, a male therapist commented on religion's ability to expand one's view of what to hope for beyond the singular hope for a child. However, in general, people who attended the monthly RESOLVE meetings seemed to appreciate the fact that RESOLVE provided a safe space that shielded them from some of the painful comments and judgments of others, including religiously based judgments.

Ethics

Only rarely did participants in the monthly meetings raise or identify any issue as a potential "ethical" problem. Once in an interview, a woman explained that she had an ethical problem with her willingness to try a procedure because her health insurance was paying for it, admitting that she probably would not have tried the procedure if she had had to pay for it herself.[87] In another interview, I asked a therapist who often led the discussion at the monthly meetings why ethical issues did not come up more often during meetings. She believed that people definitely thought about these issues—because her experience showed that they discussed such matters in individual therapy sessions—but for whatever combination of reasons, people hesitated to raise ethical issues in the group setting.[88]

Part of the ethos of RESOLVE meetings—probably reflective of some aspects of our larger society—is a generalized respect for difference and diversity. This respect extended to differences of ethical opinion or perspective.[89] I found evidence of this respect in such statements as "Everybody's different." Individuals often coupled these disclaimers of respect with more tentative statements expressing normative views. For example, one woman shared her view of adoption but then quickly qualified it: "But in a way I guess I wish people could open their hearts to children that don't have parents, but then you know everybody is different, and I don't want to visit my feelings on someone else."[90]

Two therapists who addressed RESOLVE meetings and led discussions shared their opinions in interviews. One male pastoral counselor explained his role as providing a "nonanxious presence" to his clients facing infertility: "My perspective is not to tell people what to do. They don't need someone to do that but just to help them dialogue about their decision making and hope they make good faithful choices. And I really respect the couple's decision to do that. However, there are some people who come to me and say, 'What should I do?' And I say, 'Well, that's not my job.'"[91] He did not elaborate on his definition of a "good faithful choice" or how it could be recognized. A female therapist expressed her view of the importance of mutuality in couples' decision making about infertility: "I think everybody goes about it in a different way. How you get there, I don't know. I can say how [my husband and I] got there. I guess what I look at is it has to be a mutually agreed upon thing, or later on down the road, there's too much resentment."[92]

Underneath the more explicit group norm that moral judgments from either "religious" or "ethical" sources are unhelpful lies not necessarily a lack of moral standards in decision making but a clear respect for difference. This respect is based on the fundamental assumption that decisions about infertility are regarded as highly personal or private. Ethical issues associated with these choices are also regarded as personal or private; they do not rise to the level of collective or societal concern. For whatever reasons, the members of the group were often reluctant or even afraid to identify their values (for example, mutuality between husband and wife is a good thing, adopting children who need homes is a good thing and perhaps preferable to ART, making a "faithful choice" is a good thing and looks like X). In the next chapter, I will address this reluctance to use normative language and to engage substantive ethical issues.

Examples: Egg Donation and Disclosure to Children

Inspired by the significant scholarship—particularly the work of feminists—that exists in the area of reproductive ethics, I used my research with RESOLVE as an opportunity to examine the larger social context in which decisions to use ART take place, including both cultural values such as pronatalism (aimed mainly at women) and consumerism (also involving women as the primary consumers of ART), as well as social-structural constraints such as the competing demands of work and family and the pressures of modern corporate capitalism that encourage overwork and delayed childbearing. My fieldwork also provided the opportunity to test some normative assumptions about parenthood and the importance of embodiment, or biological ties to one's offspring, especially as these assumptions interact with an "ideology of choice" and the presumptive procreative liberty discussed in chapter 1. As I attended meetings, I sought to determine whether any ethical concerns might challenge an individual couple's procreative liberty or if the group simply respected "choice" for choice's sake.

Two particular meetings helped to illustrate all of these themes in a concrete way. One dealt with the use of donor eggs, sperm, and surrogacy ("The Medical, Legal, and Emotional Aspects of Using Donor Egg or Sperm or Surrogate," April 2001). The other addressed whether and when to disclose to children the nature of their origins if they were conceived through any type of ART, particularly third-party gamete donation ("Disclosure: How Do We Tell Our Child/Children?," May 2001). The majority of speakers at both meetings focused heavily on egg donation rather than sperm donation or surrogacy, although comparisons frequently occurred between adoption and third-party donation during the second meeting on disclosure.

"The Last Opportunity"

"Our patients are usually at the last opportunity, so a lot is riding on it," explained a female physician representing a successful Atlanta-area clinic who addressed the RESOLVE group on the topic of egg donation.[93] Egg donation is a collaborative and more expensive form of ART, usually considered only when IVF with a woman's own eggs is not possible or when previous IVF cycles have not produced a viable pregnancy.[94] For women who want the experience of pregnancy and children genetically related to their husbands, egg donation is often the only option. Fortunately, because the quality of donated eggs is very good, pregnancy rates are exceptionally high; as a result, according to the physician, "This kind of work [is] so rewarding."[95]

Egg donation is a practice by and for women, by which I mean that women provide the needed eggs and other women use them. It is the inverse of gestational surrogacy, where the intended mother provides the egg and another woman (the hired surrogate) provides nine months of gestation. In the case of egg donation, the intended mother experiences pregnancy but uses an egg from someone else (the hired egg donor). She has no genetic connection to her child. Despite these differences, many feminists have criticized both practices for their potentially exploitative effects on all of the women involved. Women—or at least women with financial resources—can achieve the goal of motherhood through egg donation or surrogacy (occasionally both) but do so through highly medicalized and mediated processes. Some feminists have argued that these processes exact too high a toll on women physically, financially, psychologically, and even politically. For example, women who use egg donors give up a biological connection to their children that their husbands/partners do not (unless a sperm donor is also used). Women who use surrogates give up the experience of pregnancy. Egg donors, conversely, subject themselves to increased health risks, some of which are significant, for relatively modest financial compensation. Similarly, women who serve as surrogates accept all the risks and inconveniences of pregnancy but give the child away for pay. Their nine months of labor and their physical (and typically emotional) investment in the fetus are commodified and sold, a distortion of the reproductive process that some have argued is inherently exploitative.[96]

Egg donation, like surrogacy, may be a good example of what Rayna Rapp characterizes as "stratified reproduction."[97] This term describes, in part, the disconnection of the physical and social aspects of reproduction and parenting. Both egg donation and surrogacy are collaborative practices in the sense that more than one woman must collaborate with the provider of sperm as well as medical doctors, lab technicians, and nurses to make the pregnancy happen. More specifically, "stratified reproduction" also describes the different social locations that the various participants in these collaborative processes occupy. For example, it is likely that the hiring/intended mother in a surrogacy arrangement will be of a higher socioeconomic class than the surrogate she hires. So too are the users of egg donation likely to be more financially secure—and often older—than the egg donors they hire. Egg donation is an elite subpractice within the already elite world of assisted reproduction; it is not something that is widely available to infertile women generally. Many of the earliest feminist responses claimed that none of the women involved in these practices would benefit as greatly as the medical establishment itself. The profit to be gained and arguably the power and control exercised over biological reproduction by physicians would undermine women's agency in reproductive decisions.

Despite ethical concerns and despite its considerable extra expense, the practice of egg donation is gaining popularity in the United States. Participants at RESOLVE meetings were also far more likely to discuss egg donation than surrogacy, although egg donation was not generally considered a first-choice option. Perhaps the best explanation for egg donation's relative popularity is its high likelihood of success for older women, a sizable subset of women who use ART. At the meeting where representatives from an area clinic discussed egg donation, the physician explained that when people ask her, "Why are you so busy?" she always responds that people are waiting longer to get pregnant—"That's probably the biggest reason."[98] When the clinic's staff psychologist addressed the group, she similarly referred to the impact of a woman's age: "You can relax [when you make the decision to use a donor egg]. The biological clock isn't ticking anymore because the age of your eggs doesn't matter."[99]

These kinds of comments, which frequently infused discussions about ART, highlight an interesting mix of expectations and assumptions about women in American society generally. For example, the expectation that women naturally desire pregnancy/motherhood coexists comfortably, if paradoxically, alongside the assumption that many women are delaying childbearing to the point where they are no longer able to conceive on their own. The competing desires of motherhood and career were assumed to represent the status quo for women, and egg donation was assumed to provide a logical and appealing solution to the problem of the biological clock. In addition, the expectation that couples desire a child of "their own" coexists comfortably, if paradoxically, alongside the assumption that a donor egg still allows people to achieve their dream. Finally, this group assumed a natural order of progression in dealing with infertility in which donor eggs were considered before ART was abandoned altogether. To view egg donation as the "last opportunity" suggests that, while not ideal, many women believe that the experience of pregnancy using someone else's egg is worth having.

Two Types of Donors

In addition to the assumptions about women who need and want donor eggs, participants at RESOLVE meetings made some interesting assumptions about egg donors themselves. The psychologist who spoke to the group in April 2001 spent a long time on the process of donor selection, which involves a thorough psychological screening followed by an equally thorough medical screening. The entire time she discussed this topic, she displayed a photograph of four beautiful and healthy looking women standing in a line, smiling. The one in clearest focus was a blond with blue eyes. All of the donors had perfectly clear skin, straight white teeth, even features—obviously models.

The psychologist explained to the group that donors generally fall into two categories. The first are moms—women who chose not to have a career, who "veered off that path early on," but who have a track record of "demonstrated fertility," feel good about mothering, and now want to do something special for someone else. The second are young women who may not have partners but who have a lot of schooling ahead of them and who think they might someday need donated eggs. According to the psychologist, members of this group tend to have a strong sense of volunteerism.

It was not clear why the speaker felt that categorizing the donors was useful. Perhaps she thought it would humanize the women doing the donating and make them seem more familiar to the RESOLVE group. Maybe she even assumed that some women in the audience would identify with the second type of donor. Perhaps the categorization helped her to make sense of people's motives and to find them trustworthy. I found this casual categorization of donors to be fascinating and revealing. It is striking for its unstated, simplistic assumptions about what women in our society can do and therefore who they are. Most basically, it assumes that only discrete or mutually exclusive paths are open to women, despite all the gains in women's employment over the past few decades, and that women typically choose one path or the other. Either women work / have careers or they stay home, but their choice directly and predictably affects their childbearing decisions—both those of the women who contemplate donating eggs and those of the women who contemplate using donated eggs. The practice of egg donation thus highlights and may even reinforce what many people see as natural tracks for women in American society.

Having the "Right" Motivations

A major part of donor selection involves making sure the women have the "right" motivations for donating. The group did not discuss the recipients' motives for wanting to use a donor egg. Those motives were already assumed to be settled or at least could be discussed in the context of couples or individual therapy if any problems existed. Psychological screening precedes medical screening for donors. However, the reverse order holds true for recipients. Recipients first undergo thorough medical screening, then receive mandatory "pre-conception counseling," which includes such issues as how the couple would handle a multiple-birth pregnancy and whether the parents intend to disclose the donation to the child. There was no sense in which recipients would be evaluated for their "fitness" to be parents. On the contrary, there was a sense that this was a buyer's market and that only the sellers' goods (or the sellers themselves) would be closely scrutinized.

The psychologist described the process of selecting egg donors as quite rigorous: "I'm pretty conservative in picking donors. I want this to be a positive experience for them." They must "have interests and activities [so] that this is not their life." She administers a psychological test that examines a person's level of openness. If the testing shows that a person is "too well defended," that raises questions about the woman's credibility. "The psychological test is so important for our comfort level," explained the physician. "We really want to know that people are going through it for the right reasons, the right motivations, and don't have some underlying psychological disorder." She was looking, she said, for people with "character."[100]

"Character" seemed to mean that the prospective donor was not motivated solely by the money. Compensation for donating eggs was about five thousand dollars at this clinic,[101] and potential donors are asked directly how they plan to use the money. To help weed out women motivated only by money, donors are invited to a seminar run by the nurses at this clinic. In the seminar, potential donors learn about the full extent of the process of donating eggs, which "turns people away who are only driven by the money." Those who stay through the entire process "have a good heart."[102]

Age and weight are also important factors in choosing an egg donor. Donor women are usually aged between twenty-one and thirty-two, although some clinics have a cutoff at age thirty. The best age for donors tends to be between twenty-four and twenty-six, but the presenters did not elaborate why, and no one asked. Donors must have two functioning ovaries, cannot be smokers, and cannot be overweight. The reason cited for the weight restriction was ease of retrieval—doctors have difficulty accessing the ovaries of overweight women— but the physician also commented that obesity is not consistent with being an "appropriate candidate." Donors are required to fill out a very detailed "profile sheet" that asks "Why are you doing this?" and "Do you have any messages for the recipient couple?" The questionnaire asks prospective donors to specify their level of education, "which tends to be important to recipients."

As best as I could determine, "generosity" and "volunteerism," combined with a healthy psychological profile, constituted the "right reasons" for donating eggs, at least in the eyes of the operators of this clinic. Clinic staff expressed little willingness to explore the moral values underneath these reasons and little interest in exploring what other factors make women appropriate candidates (for example, intelligence, beauty, thinness, race, and so forth) and what moral values underlie those factors. This inability to examine or even to name the clinic's moral values raised my suspicions, primarily because I view the decision to use an egg donor as significant—for the present and future health and well-being of the donor, the recipient couple, and any resulting children.[103]

In Georgia, the clinic screens the donors on the recipient's behalf.[104] Couples are not legally permitted to meet their anonymous donors face to face or even to see a picture of their donors, although in California, recipients and anonymous donors are "meeting for lunch." The presenters praised California's leadership in many areas of the egg donation process. According to speakers at this RESOLVE meeting, 85 percent of people needing a donated egg "go the anonymous route," which takes a "little leap of faith" because the selection process is in the hands of the clinic. Known ("compassionate") donors (such as sisters or cousins) are used less often, but egg donor programs are generally more lenient about the age of the donor if she is a relative of the person using the donated egg.

Couples Must Be "on the Same Page"

Again and again I heard the advice that couples must be "on the same page" in making major decisions about their infertility. The couple needed to be in basic agreement, both for the health of their relationship and so that they could remain unified in the face of external judgments. This assumption contained a deep moral relativism that was never explored: in other words, it is less important what a couple chooses—egg donor or no egg donor, disclosure to child or not—as long as they choose together.

One of the presenters at the meeting on disclosure to children claimed that prospective parents must agree because "it can affect so much," including their marriage, their personal lives, their future children.[105] This speaker conveyed a common RESOLVE attitude toward third-party gamete donation or any form of ART: it is only a problem if one makes it a problem. For example, one participant said that using a sperm donor is "only a stigma if you make it a stigma."[106] If both parents feel good about their children's origins, the children will feel good about their origins because they pick up on their parents' cues. The fact that one parent has a biological/genetic connection that the other lacks does not necessarily have to create a problem for the marriage or for how the parents relate to their children.

Underneath these frequent references to husband and wife "needing to be on the same page" seemed to be a lingering concern about imbalances or asymmetry in a marriage relationship. However, only in the setting of an individual interview did these concerns—and a general confusion about how to proceed in decision making—find full voice:

> We really think we'll try with donor eggs. We haven't really wanted to completely make the decision until we have to. It's something that we want to be comfortable with. We're sort of not really sure how to become com-

fortable with it—what do we need to think about or how do we know if we are ready to do that or not? I'm not really sure. We started a little bit of reading on it. And it talks about some of the issues that couples face where a lot of the times the woman could end up being resentful that the husband has the genetic connection to the child and she doesn't, and we want to explore that. We want to talk to a counselor and so on because we're not going to do anything that's going to impact our relationship. We'd rather not have kids than harm our relationship in any way. But I think we'll probably get to the point that we're comfortable with that because like carrying a child, there's still a connection there. We keep saying if it was a sperm donor, that's totally different because then he would have no connection whatsoever.[107]

Her comments underscore some typical assumptions about gender differences that have already been mentioned: the experience of pregnancy somehow offsets the lack of genetic connection between mother and child, increasing people's general comfort level with donor eggs. In addition, equality between husband and wife, while very important, does not depend on both parents having the same literal connection to the resulting child. Nevertheless, this woman seemed to express uncertainty about how to draw meaningful distinctions (for example, between egg and sperm donation) and about how to reach a final decision. The public RESOLVE meetings did not seem likely to provide her with a setting in which she could deeply explore her questions, and she noted that she and her husband were already reading and deliberating together.

"It Doesn't Matter Where the Egg Comes From"

Both the presenters and the participants/interviewees seemed to agree that "it doesn't matter where the egg comes from." Since one presenter entirely skipped the "ethical issues" section of her presentation, noting that when a third-party donor is used, couples primarily concern themselves with whether to disclose the donation to their children, it seems plausible to surmise that creating a child from an anonymous donor egg does not in itself raise ethical issues. However, I wondered whether the meeting really made available a space in which participants could raise ethical concerns. For example, the physician claimed that couples' questions usually center on emotional, psychological, and/or financial aspects of the egg donor process. From her standpoint as a physician, she said, "We can provide all the medical information and support you through the process."[108] But by defining the boundaries of concern in this way, she seemed to close the door on other kinds of problems or questions.

The presenters claimed that donors have no attachment to what they are donating, that it is more like donating blood than giving up a baby. When asked by the group about the psychological impact of disclosure on the resulting children, some of the presenters at the May 2001 meeting admitted that the studies were "just not there yet" because children born through this process are not yet teenagers. Presenters at the April 2001 meeting with clinic representatives vaguely referred to European studies of the effects of egg donation on children that found no differences between the donor group, in which the donation was not disclosed to the child, and the control group, in which both parents were biologically related to the child. There were no problems of attachment. "Egg donation did not feel psychologically relevant as time went on."[109]

A personal presentation by one of the copresidents and her husband corroborated these claims. Their child, a toddler at the time, had been conceived with an egg donated by the wife's sister. They reported that the donation "was a very open and celebrated thing" among their families, and that if any family members had had a problem with their decision to use an egg donor, it "was interesting they had that opinion but not relevant," according to the husband. The wife's sister was a "special aunt," but not in a "weird or possessive way." Echoing the European study, they reported that the donation became less and less relevant over time: their daughter was theirs. Their biggest challenge, as they saw it, was finding a way to convey the story of her origins over time. But the key was to convey that it was a positive story and to express to the child that she was loved.[110]

In fact, most of the group's discussion seemed to focus on the issue of disclosure. Participants were concerned about teaching children enough science so that they could comprehend how they were created. Others were more interested in keeping the donation confidential, to protect the child's privacy. The general advice seemed to be that if parents plan to tell a lot of people, they must first tell the children, because it can be very "damaging" for them to find out from someone else. Moreover, "You don't want to wait until the child is a teenager, because there are so many identity issues that children have in their teens." Parents should start introducing the idea early on, in age-appropriate ways, and keep the explanation simple and matter-of-fact—for example, "A kind lady gave Mommy an egg." Again, without much substantiation, the staff psychologist from the clinic claimed that being a child of a donated egg/sperm is different from adoption: "Sharing eggs is different from coming to terms with the fact that someone relinquished you as a baby."[111]

My interviews also seemed to support my impression that women were not overly concerned with the egg donation itself. For example, one woman who briefly considered using a donor egg after a miscarriage with her own egg stated, "Somehow being pregnant . . . made me realize it doesn't matter where the egg comes from."[112] Another woman who was contemplating using a donor egg said, "I've talked to some people about [using a donor egg] that have done it, and they say it's—once you carry the child, . . . you just stop thinking about it eventually and it's your child."[113] The first of these two women chose to adopt rather than go through with the egg donation; the second expressed considerable ambivalence and still had not reached a firm decision when I concluded my research.

"Would You Have Wanted Your Parents to Tell You?"

Since disclosure is viewed as the primary ethical issue facing couples who use third-party donors, it seemed fitting that the presenter for that meeting asked group members a question to get them thinking critically: "Put yourself in the child's shoes. If you were born from donor eggs or sperm, would you have wanted your parents to tell you?" She then advised them to find out as much medical information about their donors as possible so that they would be able to provide that information to the child. She was straightforward about her starting premise: disclosure is preferable to secrecy.

The group members talked about their experiences with adoption, trying to forge analogies with egg/sperm donation. Some of the participants talked about growing up with adopted siblings, while some had worked with adopted children. All reported a great appreciation for adopted children's desire to know about their biological origins and the difficulties that can arise when that information is kept from them. In one case, two brothers had been adopted through Catholic Social Services and no information was available. In another case, the parents hid a box of information about their adopted child and would not share it with him.

At the earlier meeting, one participant had raised the question of gaining access to donors' identities. The clinic physician assured the questioner that identities are coded and kept under lock and key for emergency access. Donors are asked if their identities may be revealed for future medical reasons. When the woman followed up by asking what would happen if the clinic ever closed, the physician assured her that would never happen.

Group members seemed to have some obvious anxiety about disclosure issues as well as the closely related issues of stigma and notoriety from egg/sperm donation. One of the RESOLVE leaders reassuringly told the group members that she believed that over the next five to ten years, as these technologies become more common and accepted, using donors would be "less taboo." In fact, she explicitly cited deferred childbearing: as more people waited to have children, more people would consider the use of these technologies as an option. Adoption went from being almost always closed to almost always open, she noted. Use of donors would probably be the same.[114]

Review of Norms Identified

RESOLVE discussions, taken as a whole, created an ethos with recognizable norms. Some of these norms pertained to the organization itself: for example, what the organization says it stands for, what is appropriate to say or not say at meetings, who is invited to speak at meetings, who feels welcome to attend meetings, what may be printed in the local newsletter, and so forth. These norms defined the boundaries of the space and what makes this organization unique or at least distinguishable from other organizations such as Hannah's Prayer, a Christian support group for infertility, or other groups, clubs, or for-profit clinics.

Some of the norms concerned how to cope with infertility: for example, how to manage one's feelings and generally take care of oneself, how to handle comments from family and friends, how to stay in communication with one's spouse, and how to proceed toward resolution. Proceeding toward resolution often followed a predictable ordering of options: first low-tech treatment, then high-tech treatment, then consideration of using a third-party donor (if applicable), then a consideration of adoption. These norms defined the boundaries and contours of the process of dealing with infertility and how this particular group interpreted what was important in that process, including practical matters such as the medical, legal, and financial aspects of treatment or adoption.

A final area concerned more controversial ethical issues or problems. These so-called private decisions included whether to use a third-party gamete donor, whether both parents should share a genetic as well as social connection to their child, whether to disclose to children that they were created from donors, when to stop treatment,[115] and many others. The norm that generally governed these decisions was respect for different opinions or for procreative liberty and freedom of choice. At the heart of these issues or problems, the group rightly recognized, lay the content of people's most fundamental values and beliefs.

However, even here in the area of private conscience, the group had tentative, emergent norms. For example, the group felt there should be no stigma in using ART, including third-party donors, there should be no stigma in adoption, and there should be no stigma in childlessness. Moreover, openness or disclosure was generally judged to be better than secrecy, and mutuality in partnership or marriage was judged superior to disagreement or unilateral decision making. Despite the uncritical acceptance of a "natural" desire to have a child of "one's own" through ART or to match traits and race if using a third-party donor, group members generally seemed to believe that children are valuable for who they are and not the process by which they got here or the particular traits they possess. In other words, biological origins mattered up front, at the stage of conception, but receded in importance as a bond with an actual child was forged, whether through birth or adoption. Many group members ultimately did not care where the egg—or the child—came from. Finally, and perhaps even more paradoxically, the group generally embraced the idea that people should not be consumed by their infertility (and their infertility treatments) to the point where they forget the value of their wider life—even in the midst of undergoing treatment.

These norms were generally easy to find, although doing so sometimes required looking beyond the explicit assertions of neutrality or freedom of opinion and choice. In the next chapter, I will take a more critical look at RESOLVE's assertions of nonjudgmental support and the priority given to freedom of choice. A paramount consideration is whether the participants in the group meetings possessed the resources and vocabulary to challenge the subtle (and sometimes not so subtle) pressures to consume these technologies, pressures I believe were reinforced by the clinic representatives and physicians who addressed the group.

FOUR

Contributions from Ethics

Gender, Consumerism, and Challenges
to the Ethos of Neutrality

The Conversation

When I examined more closely the substance of the conversations that took place at RESOLVE's public monthly meetings, both by reviewing my field notes and reflecting on my accumulated experience with this particular group, it was evident that RESOLVE members and leaders often lacked a critical engagement with any larger context beyond the individual and immediate goal of having a baby. Generally speaking, people did not question the broader implications of private choices or how those choices were shaped by forces outside of the individual's or couple's desires.

One area that illustrates this lack of engagement with a larger context was the group's tendency to import gendered expectations about the use of assisted reproductive technologies (ART) and gendered scripts for the experience of infertility without seriously questioning those scripts. Participants evidenced little or no sustained interest in the idea of pronatalism and whether it fuels the use of ART, for example. Nor did group members consider whether delayed childbearing and its associated social-structural problems might unfairly burden women.

Group members also failed to challenge the subtle and not-so-subtle pressures to consume ART, pressures that clinic representatives and physicians who addressed the group often reinforced. Any inclination participants might have had to criticize American habits of consumption with regard to ART was routinely overwhelmed by the desire to become educated, proactive consumers who made cost-effective choices. Group members also avoided explicitly reflecting on socioeconomic class and its role in using ART.

By focusing on the themes of gender and consumerism in this chapter—both what was said and not said in group discussions—I challenge RESOLVE's ethos of neutrality, its pervasive emphasis on nonjudgmental support and freedom of choice. While this ethos seemingly supported individuals in their decision making, the rhetoric of moral neutrality and respect for "private" choices also contributed to the overall lack of engagement with a larger context, including but not limited to issues of gender justice and consumerism. This observation tends to confirm Lisa Cahill's point that absent a critical conversation examining the final ends of ART, the ability to see any connection between social-structural forces and individual choices is greatly diminished.

Important reasons exist for seeing this connection between private choices and larger contexts. Not only does a certain blindness to larger contexts, including whether people are making truly free and informed decisions, affect the moral agency of decision makers, but it also impacts, in a more general sense, human flourishing and the common good. For example, the group's absorption in the task of achieving pregnancy created costly vulnerabilities for people stuck on the "treadmill of infertility." Since RESOLVE's self-described mission is advocacy for the infertile, I believe it is appropriate and fair to appraise that mission in light of these vulnerabilities. How well does RESOLVE protect the interests of the infertile? Rather than unconditional validation of private choices, we need richer publics and more critical conversations.

Finally, while focusing on the themes of gender and consumerism, I discuss where the relevant scholarship on these points has been valid and helpful as well as where I have found it overly simplistic or lacking in nuance. This critique of theory in light of observations about a social world embodies my overarching goal of letting experience speak to ethics.

Gender Differences and Gendered Expectations

Aging Eggs and the Market for ART

As I discussed in chapter 3, conversations at RESOLVE meetings undeniably contained a subtext about gender. Participants had an implicit—or in some cases explicit—awareness of a larger social context with regard to gender, but this awareness often had a taken-for-granted quality, as something beyond the concern or control of individual decision makers. For example, discussion leaders and participants frequently noted that more and more women now use ART because many people are choosing to delay childbearing while pursuing careers. Not only was this reason for using ART accepted uncritically as the status quo, but discussion leaders suggested on a number of occasions that the trends of delayed childbearing and ART use would only increase. The result, they predicted, would be greater societal acceptance of ART procedures, including the use of donor eggs and surrogacy, less secrecy about the decisions, less secrecy in the selection of donors, and more resources (for example, children's books and psychological studies) to help children adjust to the knowledge of their origins. These developments were deemed positive, especially by the clinic representatives who specialized in egg donation but also by experienced RESOLVE leaders and counselors—people who gave every impression of having their fingers on the pulse of our culture's views of assisted reproduction. The reason for their optimism: greater societal acceptance of ART promises more choices for aspiring parents and reduced stigma for their potential children.[1]

The general acceptance of delayed childbearing as a cultural reality in the present and future and as a notable departure from the past lent an air of unqualified acceptance to ART procedures that specifically solve the problem of aging eggs. If some women in the group regretted that their increased freedom to pursue a career had come at the price of diminished fertility, no one lingered long on this unhappy thought. The group's approach was fundamentally pragmatic: How can we fix age-related infertility, given the fact that the biological clock ticks more loudly for women than men? Egg donation is one of the best solutions currently available to older women in terms of likelihood of producing a viable pregnancy, but other procedures on the horizon, including egg freezing or banking, promise more options in the future.[2] At none of the meetings I attended did participants or leaders raise concerns about the safety of more experimental procedures. People at the "Ask the Experts" meeting expressed curiosity about cytoplasmic transfer, but because it is not widely available, the level of interest in discussing it was low.

Some of the discussion leaders—usually the physicians—were willing to raise concerns about the more experimental ART procedures and openly criticized what they perceived as the irresponsible use of some procedures known to have low success rates for older women.[3] These physicians articulated that their motivation to restrict certain uses of ART was based on a professional duty to protect the health of their patients, not a desire to limit freedom of choice or even to maximize clinics' success rates. Other physicians, however—most notably the entrepreneurial doctor/Internet consultant who visited RESOLVE to discuss how to distinguish valuable information from "garbage" on the Internet and to advertise his Web site—seemed more than happy to turn decisions over to the free market and to rational, self-educated choosers. His approach was less paternalistic and more laissez-faire: he was interested in giving the people what they wanted, whatever that was, and providing his clients with cutting-edge services. (He did, however, joke that a computer keyboard plus an Internet chat did not equal a pelvic exam. Women still need the in-person care of their physicians, he counseled.) He was loath to concede any safety concerns—"You hear that [ART drugs] cause cancer. They don't, they don't"—let alone raise questions about societal trends fueling the consumption of ART.[4]

The RESOLVE leaders at these meetings seemed equally open to these physicians' divergent philosophies about what constitutes good medical practice. Paternalistic concerns for patients' "best interests" received equal airtime with portrayals of medical care as a commodity in a free market where patients' "rights" and "choices" are paramount. Neither participants nor leaders offered any comments about which approach does a better job of supporting the interests of the infertile. All information directed toward the goal of resolving infertility was deemed equally valid.

Even those physicians who ventured to question certain uses of ART, such as whether women in their forties or fifties ought to attempt in vitro fertilization (IVF) with their own eggs, almost always raised concerns in the context of addressing an individual question or problem rather than venturing to address a broader social issue such as delayed childbearing. They approached the discussion as individual professionals who treat individual patients. They viewed ART as the best modern medicine has to offer infertile patients, not as a potentially controversial response to the social "problem" of delayed childbearing. What seemed to be missing was the willingness to connect the personal experience of infertility with larger trends in American society and to raise any questions about the current situation or to imagine how it might be different. All participants and leaders seemed to agree that little could be gained by scrutinizing societal trends in which we are all inextricably involved and that lamenting past individual choices had even less benefit. Both were perceived as unchangeable or at least as part of an unchanging external landscape through which the individual or couple was now navigating. Many women delay childbearing, often leading to infertility: Now, how can we move forward and have a baby?

This eager focus on having children by any means necessary disturbs many ethicists, particularly feminist ethicists. More fundamentally, they are bothered by an uncritical acceptance of the legitimacy of the desire to have children. As discussed earlier, many feminists believe that ART reinforces oppressive gender roles by overemphasizing women's reproductive capacities.[5] Some feminist observers argue that expectations of technology and gender become intertwined and mutually reinforcing: pronatalism tells women they must have a baby, and technology tells them they can. Did any voices within RESOLVE question these expectations?

The gender subtext in the RESOLVE discussions included numerous comments about how the experience of infertility is "different" for women. These comments sometimes referred to the physical differences in treatment, because women undergo the majority of invasive procedures when trying to become pregnant regardless of whether there is female-factor and/or male-factor infertility. The comments at times referred to more general experiential differences, such as women's greater investment in researching and pursuing treatment options, women's different ways of coping with the disappointment of infertility, or even how the nature of the disappointment differs for women because more of their sense of self/identity is connected to relationships and mothering.[6]

Perhaps only in this last observation—that the nature of the disappointment in infertility is different for women as a consequence of their different expectations about motherhood—are Cahill and other feminists justified in their concerns about pronatalism pushing women to use ART. Cahill assumes that women will feel additional pressure to conceive children because of still-strong stereotypes that say biological parenthood is essential to women's adult identity. I certainly saw evidence to support this claim. For example, a male therapist told me in an interview, "There's nothing more feminine than giving birth."[7] But most comments by discussion participants, especially women, were less stark. No one seemed to be pursuing treatment because she believed reproduction was woman's most important purpose in life. Most women who came to RESOLVE had other "purposes" in life, including careers, schooling, and caring for existing children.

After observing women (and men) in RESOLVE, I believe that the charge of pronatalism is overly simplistic for a number of reasons. First, although the experience of child-free living was a minor story told by RESOLVE members, it was still considered a legitimate option. Some women in RESOLVE had decided that their lives were full enough without children and without the experience of biological reproduction. Most of the child-free women I met were longtime members who kept returning to meetings to testify to their experience—usually of how they had come to the decision to cease infertility treatments and then, for whatever reasons, to forgo adoption. In the context of the monthly meetings, there was room enough for choosing not to parent any children, and that choice was supported, even if it remained the less traveled path.

Second, the charge of pronatalism—that women internalize an overpowering message from society that they cannot be complete without the experience of pregnancy and childbirth—obscures the relevant factors of delayed childbearing and what some sociologists have described as a changed understanding of middle-class selfhood. For example, in *The Fabric of Self* (1998), Diane Margolis argues that American society may be experiencing a relatively new understanding of middle-class selfhood, the construction of which is tied closely to work and career identity for both women and men, in contrast to previous generations. In this new understanding of selfhood, childbearing may be delayed to accommodate greater expectations for the self and self-development. Essayist Katha Pollitt also points out that pursuing other life goals while not focusing on, insisting on, or prioritizing having children is a way of choosing not to have children and that there is nothing wrong with this choice.[8] She seeks to encourage women to take ownership of the decision to delay childbearing, conscious or not, and then to accept, without too much regret, what that choice says about the legitimacy of pursuing other life goals. She reminds us that childlessness need not be viewed as a "tragic blunder."

Although it could be easily argued that women who delay childbearing remain deeply influenced by pronatalism—they want children as much or perhaps more than women who do not delay—the charge of pronatalism seems too one-dimensional to capture the series of complex decisions and trade-offs that can lead to the use of ART. A more accurate or nuanced assessment, based on what women who use ART say and do, may not focus exclusively on attacking the drive to have children as illegitimate but rather look at the desire for children as one important drive among many others. Feminist theologian Bonnie Miller-McLemore has written about the concept of generativity, which she defines as both contributing to the wider world through work and caring for persons through parenting.[9] She argues that both women and men have generative needs but that society tends to value and support only "productivity," which is a truncated version of generativity. She writes, "Social structures that reward those who produce and penalize those who take care preclude full actualization of generativity for both men and women."[10] If one takes seriously the generative drive of women to fulfill both productive and reproductive goals, one is less likely to view ART and the quest for children as an obvious cause of women's oppression.[11] Since I take these drives seriously, I am not ready to dismiss ART as hopelessly oppressive or the pursuit of motherhood as a sign that women do not know what it is they want and need when they seek treatment for infertility.

Rather than focus on the desire for children as itself somehow defective, the critique should perhaps more reasonably and compassionately be directed elsewhere. For example, given all the ways society could respond to the bodily realities of pregnancy, childbirth, and the primary care of small children, our society continually re-creates social structures that make these realities especially burdensome to women. We should scrutinize not individual women's choices but our democratic society's commitment to equality and social justice—or, more specifically, how our society might better support the work of reproducing the next generation. In addition, one could look at whether people perceive a technology such as ART as compensating for bodily differences between men and women insofar as ART helps to extend the biological clock for women. (Those who would market the "career pill" and egg freezing surely play on this hope.) To examine our expectations of technology in this way shifts the focus of what counts as the problem: it is not necessarily pronatalism by itself but rather our naive expectation that technology can bypass embodied limitations and social-structural problems.

However, pronatalism may still accurately capture part of the problem in one sense: it preys on women's tendency to blame themselves for their infertility. In RESOLVE meetings, women often expressed feelings of being punished for waiting too long, for trying to combine career and family aspirations, and for doing things differently than their mothers or sisters. Pronatalism may validate this perception of punishment: it encourages the idea that women who dare to prioritize other life goals have abnegated the higher duty of motherhood. People in the meetings I observed generally pushed back against this idea, with the fervent help of discussion leaders and therapists. These women were encouraged to express their anger at the unfairness and arbitrariness of infertility. After all, they only wanted what the "fertile world" already has, not more. Still, these women seemed particularly vulnerable to experiencing their infertility as punishment, which may have motivated them to try ART and willingly and repeatedly to endure its discomforts and disappointments.

Indeed, one way to interpret the treadmill metaphor used so frequently by RESOLVE members to refer to successive trials of IVF may be that many women approach ART as something akin to an ascetic ritual.[12] To the extent that women have borrowed time to pursue other life goals in their twenties and thirties, they may feel that some payment is due, perhaps in the form of an exacting regimen of drug therapies and medical procedures. When people talked about the "treadmill of ART," they very clearly had the exercise machine in mind. Their workout was not pursued for enjoyment but for the long-term payoff of a baby. In the interpretation of ART as an ascetic ritual, the exigencies of repeated treatments would also be endured as payment (or punishment) for a prior indulgence.

On the whole, despite the obvious influence of pronatalism, this explanation needs to be nuanced. The charge of pronatalism by itself provides too easy an excuse for dismissing a group such as RESOLVE, as if the only factor were the single-minded pursuit of babies. Such a pursuit unquestionably occurred, but it does not speak to the personal transformation process that is the focus of the next chapter, the extent to which truly "resolving" one's infertility often comes to include more complex goals than simply getting a baby. Reducing the desires of infertile individuals who seek out the support of fellow RESOLVE members to pronatalism also diverts attention away from the group's self-described mission of advocacy for the interests of the infertile, which could theoretically include many interests beyond having a baby, and ignores the question of how well RESOLVE is achieving that mission. Such a simplification ultimately discredits the full extent of the support RESOLVE in fact provides its members. The pressures of pronatalism surely explain some of the use of ART, but it is not the whole story.

Structural Constraints on Women's Choices: Work and Family

As stated earlier, I am concerned that ART might encourage women to delay childbearing. This use of ART concerns me because I believe such a technological fix constitutes an insufficient response to unjust social structures that make it difficult for women to fulfill various generative needs within a lifespan of typical length. My research with RESOLVE focused on the impact of work/family conflicts on women's decisions to use ART: I listened for this theme in the group conversations and asked questions about it in my individual interviews.[13] I have suggested that pronatalism (the coercive societal message that motherhood or parenthood is essential to adult identity), while important, does not fully illuminate the larger context of individuals' decisions to use ART. Do work/family conflicts shed more light on the phenomenon of increasing ART use?

The discussions I observed at RESOLVE meetings did not contain nearly the level of explicit concern about work/family conflicts that I brought to this project as a researcher. Yet although discussion participants did not describe or categorize their concerns using the language of "work/family conflicts" or "structural constraints," the realities of work and family life in the twenty-first-century United States framed many conversations. Leaders and presenters often drew on certain scripts for women with regard to work and family choices, and participants generally accepted these scripts without challenge. One of the best examples, mentioned in the preceding chapter, was a clinic representative's pat explanation of the two types of egg donors—stay-at-home moms wanting to do something generous and important, and young aspiring professionals with a sense of volunteerism and a hunch that they may someday need donated eggs.[14] The psychologist's typologies stirred no controversy and elicited no questions from the audience. She was merely reporting an interesting fact, something fairly obvious to her but worth pointing out to the uninitiated, perhaps as a way to give a human face to the anonymous women undergoing major medical procedures to donate their genetic material to strangers. In no way did she suggest that these two types warranted concern.

Despite her ostensible agenda of neutral reporting, from another perspective, the psychologist was conveying her clinic's moral values about who makes a good donor. Not just anyone can be a donor (for example, the clinic does not accept overweight women as donors), and not just anyone should be. The clinic representative considered money a poor motivation for donating but approved of generosity or volunteerism as a motivator. Perhaps this psychologist found women in these two categories acceptable egg donors because they represented appropriate categories for women generally: either women have children, or women have a career. The psychologist probably knew she could count on her audience to share these culturally determined, gender-specific expectations about work and family.

The unstated message in the psychologist's sketch seems to be that women who stay at home with their children would obviously crave taking on an important and more public project such as donating their eggs to someone who needs them. The desire to donate in this situation makes sense because these women have not been denied the opportunity to have children of their own but may not have had the chance to contribute to something outside their families. It is morally acceptable, even laudable, to give generously in this way.

The unstated message for women who choose to pursue education and careers seems to be that of course they would be unable to have children until much later, possibly when they are no longer fertile. So again, the desire to donate makes sense, especially when paired with the self-interested motive of supplying eggs to a clinic that may someday service the donor. Nothing is going to change to make it any easier for women to combine careers with family—nor, necessarily, should it—so why not give generously now and take what one needs later?[15]

These are limited possibilities to imagine for women—two mutually exclusive tracks. The taken-for-granted naturalness of these tracks or forced choices explains, I believe, why the clinic's psychologist thought it self-evident that egg donors would generally come from one or the other of these two pools and why no one in the RESOLVE group that night thought her categorization was particularly significant. I disagree. Why do we still accept the background assumption that women must choose between work and family, as if these were the only two major alternatives in a zero-sum game? What difference would it make for the conversation if someone suggested that the zero-sum game could be rewritten more fairly?

RESOLVE's literature indicated that other organization members had considered these questions, too. For example, the *Managing Friends and Family* pamphlet offered instructions to the infertile for dealing with associates who asked, "When are you going to stop concentrating on your career and start a family?" The suggested response defends, without apology, the legitimacy of combining work and family: "I don't believe my job and family are mutually exclusive. My career is advancing, and I'm very happy with my work. When we feel the time is right, we will consider starting our family." This confident reply, however inspiring it might have been for members to read, was not at all representative of the mood at meetings.

As I have already discussed, many participants in group discussions commented on working and deferred childbearing, and many of these statements were comparative comments about how other women choose differently. There was a notable sense of competition and envy among women, including between a boss and her subordinate employee who was pregnant, between sisters and sisters-in-law, and between mothers and daughters who made different choices in life. Most significant in these comments was the refrain of frustration turned inward, to an interpersonal level, rather than outward, to social structures. Such statements accented personal choices and consequences, displaying a tendency to internalize or personalize rather than to explore the idea of individual actors caught up in a web of social forces. I believe that in fostering more critical reflection about society rather than encouraging self-blame, certain ethical perspectives can become valuable contributors to the conversation about ART.

Theories of social justice are particularly useful in understanding the larger context in which we find ourselves and the choices that we believe are available to us. They fall short, however, of addressing all of the ethical issues raised by ART. Not all of what is significant about why increasing numbers of people use ART can be attributed to delayed childbearing or to the pressures of combining work and family goals. My research with RESOLVE has helped me to recognize my biases and to put the work / family problem in perspective. I still believe that feminist arguments about the "deflective" power of ART have merit: it may well be, as Laura A. Woliver and Dorothy Roberts claim, that the availability of this technological fix deflects efforts to make more substantial and long-lasting changes toward sexual equality.[16] Yet these arguments need to be nuanced. Even more than the charge of pronatalism, the characterization of ART as a technological fix oversimplifies the complex desires and intentions of individual choosers, people making decisions with tangible consequences. Upon reflection, perhaps the most useful idea we can take from these theories is more modest: an uncritical acceptance of these limited possibilities for women is disempowering by itself and should be challenged wherever possible.

Susan Moller Okin and the many feminists who have built on her ideas are helpful for imagining how social structures might be different.[17] In her now-classic text, *Justice, Gender, and the Family* (1989), Okin argues that a more just society would begin with a more just family, where mothers and fathers share equally in parenthood. Her goal is to move beyond gendered roles and expectations so that women are not systematically disadvantaged as society's presumptive caregivers. Her most practical suggestion is the creation of a family workweek in which parents together work no more than sixty hours total, staggering their schedules so that they can share child care when it is not provided by high-quality day care centers or other sources.[18]

A number of feminist writers, including economist Nancy Folbre and philosopher Eva Feder Kittay, have developed the argument, sometimes referred to as an "ethic of care," that a just society should not view childbearing and child rearing as merely a personal choice or source of private fulfillment but as a social activity.[19] Kittay's idea of "caring for the caregiver" provides a critique of liberal equality. She acknowledges that the Enlightenment ideal of equality has benefited women but argues that the ideal is ultimately incoherent. If equality is conceived as an association of equals (that is, heads of households), it risks obscuring the fact of dependency, the needs of dependents, and the work, both paid and unpaid, required to sustain people who are not yet fully autonomous or no longer or never capable of caring for themselves. One problem is that "progress," according to the ideal of liberal equality, requires changing only one side of the sexual division of labor: more women on the male side of productive labor. What is lacking is a fundamental restructuring of expectations of men and a rethinking of the gendered structure itself. Given that we all benefit from the rearing of children as healthy and productive citizens, society should find ways to support this activity, not penalize economically or otherwise the people who do the caregiving.[20]

Philosopher and political theorist Seyla Benhabib phrases the problem in terms of contradictions between spheres that diminish one's chances for agency in one sphere based on one's membership in another. The nature of the activities involved (for example, taking care of a baby and earning a paycheck) may make it hard to participate in both spheres. Their mutual exclusivity may then be reinforced by the system: "Take the duties of motherhood and the public aspirations of women in the economy, politics or science, and the fact that public funds are not used to support better, more readily available and more affordable forms of childcare."[21] Benhabib argues that reducing the contradictions between spheres would increase political participation; I suggest that doing so would also go a long way toward slowing the trend of delayed childbearing. Instead of pushing childbearing to the forties and beyond for professional women, all women might encounter a greater variety of options for defining and pursuing their generative goals at every stage of life.

I believe that this imaginative act—thinking about reconstructing society in a way that is more fair—frees people to think outside the narrow paths that are so often assumed to be part of the natural landscape.[22] Such an approach empowers people to question whether it is good that women delay childbearing, for example. Perhaps fathers should share more of the activity of parenting, or government should sponsor universal preschool, or workplaces should do more to curb overwork. To think about justice and fairness also gives people a sense that they can participate in shaping society. Insofar as theories of social justice encourage people to think critically about what is fair and to imagine themselves as somehow shaping a more fair society rather than passively accepting predetermined roles and expectations, these theories are relevant to and useful for analyzing the phenomenon of ART.

Whether because of the therapists, the physicians, the clinic representatives, the RESOLVE leaders, the discussion participants, or all of these factors, the conversations I observed at RESOLVE meetings unquestionably assumed an individualistic framework. They focused on how individuals can be informed consumers, savvy researchers, and wise managers of their own emotions, but these empowering messages applied only to the immediate crisis of infertility. Feminists who engage a social justice perspective, such as Okin, Folbre, Kittay, and Benhabib, look at social structures and the systemic problems they cause or exacerbate. They help us examine goals and structures beyond the individual aim of having a baby. In so doing, they widen the boundaries of the conversation, enabling it to move beyond self-blame toward an understanding of the self as part of a larger community or common good. They also open up the possibility of constructive change. I value these contributions because I value a greater sense of self-determination and of participating in and improving society's structures.

I now turn to a consideration of the impact of consumerism on the use of ART. Although I have separated issues of gender and consumerism for the purposes of discussion, I believe these issues are in reality intertwined. These forces are implicated together in questions of agency and self-determination, and a more nuanced ethical account of ART must view questions of gender justice through the powerfully structuring effects of consumerist individualism.

Class and Consumerism

The Privileges and Pressures of an Elite

A year of attendance at RESOLVE's monthly meetings might well lead an observer to believe that a great many people use high-tech assisted reproduction to become pregnant. As discussed in earlier chapters, participants in these meetings generally presumed that infertility should be treated medically, just as hypertension should be controlled with diet and exercise and cancer should be treated with chemotherapy.[23] The question was not usually whether to try IVF, for example, but how many times to try it.

One notable exception to the general belief that ART represents the commonsense answer to a common problem was the view expressed by Alice Domar, a prominent spokesperson and researcher in the field of infertility treatment, who flew to Atlanta from Boston's Mind/Body Clinic to run a "Women's Retreat" for RESOLVE in the early spring of 2001. The retreat, one of the special Saturday symposia offered during the year to paying members, was held in the sunny banquet hall of a suburban country club north of Atlanta. After some opening remarks about the relationship between stress and infertility—always a delicate topic in RESOLVE because of its implication that infertile people somehow cause their own infertility—Domar asked her audience, a group of about one hundred women, to break into smaller discussion groups. The women, already seated at round tables covered with white linen tablecloths and brightly colored centerpieces (which we later learned were RESOLVE candles wrapped in pink and orange tissue paper), received a topic to discuss. Within minutes, the room was filled with the sounds of women trading stories about infertility.

Domar walked around the room, sitting in on various conversations, and after a short while called for everyone's attention to provide what she called a "reality check." Without being accusatory, she said that the conversations gave the impression that each person thought she was *supposed* to try IVF. But, she pointed out, only half of all people experiencing infertility ever see a doctor, and only half of that group see a doctor more than once. Of those, only 2 or 3 percent attempt IVF. According to Domar, "There shouldn't be an expectation that you *should* do IVF. Most people who go through infertility don't get treatment. . . . You are pushing yourselves very hard."[24] In short, she reminded the women that the people in this country who are even considering IVF are among a very small and privileged group. She seemed to want not to make the women feel bad for their privileged location but rather to provide perspective —a "reality check"—and to encourage them to go easy on themselves, to resist feeling obligated to try this specialized treatment.

Domar's good intentions notwithstanding, it seemed a small consolation for the women at the retreat to hear that the vast majority of Americans facing infertility do not seek treatment with high-tech assisted reproduction. More immediately pressing to them was the fact that they and the people they knew were in the midst of preparing themselves physically and emotionally for cycles of ART.[25] In fact, when I talked to some of the women after the retreat, they reported that the workshops on yoga, aromatherapy, and other stress-reducing techniques had been the most useful. They liked the message of "self-care," but it was unclear whether anyone challenged the fundamental expectation that they should try at least some treatment.

Regardless of how her reality check was received, Domar's remarks stood out in my research as an unusually direct reminder of the larger universe outside the world of infertility treatments and an unusually explicit acknowledgment of the pressures experienced by an elite group of people. Her faith in ART seemed noticeably lower than that of the clinic representatives and physicians who regularly addressed RESOLVE meetings with the partial motive of attracting new patients. She was most concerned with helping women to "get their lives back" and "become the people they used to be" rather than necessarily achieving pregnancy.[26] In fact, she called pregnancy a "nice side effect" of the pursuit of overall health and the reduction of stress and depression. Her belief that aiming at health rather than directly at pregnancy can assist in treating infertility starkly contrasted with the "try as much treatment as your budget will allow" approach best exemplified by the entrepreneurial Internet doctor. Domar based her remarks on her empirical research on the relationship between depression and infertility. This research, her published books, and the Mind/Body Clinic in Boston have earned Domar a strong reputation in the field of infertility treatment. She noted that women with a history of depression are twice as likely to experience infertility: the pregnancy rate for depressed women is 13 percent, while for women who are not depressed, the pregnancy rate is 29 percent. She also explicitly questioned the ethics of starting an IVF cycle on a woman with depression.[27]

Domar approached this group of women not as potential patients (although she certainly stood to gain financially if any of them later visited her Mind/Body Clinic or another one of her retreats) but as a group of people especially vulnerable to getting stuck on the treadmill of infertility. She did not offer a simple explanation for this vulnerability but referred explicitly to its costs. She told a story about a woman in Massachusetts (a state that mandates insurance coverage for infertility treatments) who had undergone twenty-six unsuccessful IVF cycles. The audience gasped at the number, which Domar called "sick." Domar also called this woman an "exceptional case" and claimed that "most women in Massachusetts don't do more IVF because it's covered."[28]

I considered many possibilities for why this group was so vulnerable to getting stuck on the treadmill, including the role of class and race. Feminist scholars, including Rayna Rapp and Roberts, have theorized that class and race are built into the preference for assisted reproduction and that the use of ART reinforces existing economic and racial inequalities. Because most insurance plans do not cover infertility treatments, access is usually limited to those who can afford to pay out of pocket. People with the means to pay for one IVF trial out of pocket may have the ability to pay for several more, thus making them more vulnerable to continuing with unsuccessful treatments. It certainly marks a sharp divergence in the experiences of poor and wealthy infertile patients. In addition, the vast majority of infertile patients who pursue ART are white. Insofar as race is a proxy for socioeconomic status, as some demographers of ART use have suggested,[29] this observation may not carry great significance. However, other reasons, independent of wealth, may explain why whites are drawn to ART. Roberts claims that a desire for racial purity motivates white Americans to try ART rather than considering adoption. She also cites racial differences in attitudes toward technology and trust in the medical community.[30] Whites may put their faith in medical technology and may keep returning even when it fails them.

My case study primarily examined the elite group that uses ART. One of the limitations of this focus is that I did not find out how other populations experience infertility or how they feel about assisted reproduction. One of the benefits of this focus, however, was that it enabled me to examine this privileged group in greater depth—who they are, their motivations, and the sources of the pressures they experience. Class- and race-specific assumptions require greater scrutiny because, like assumptions about gender, they are often presupposed in the conversation with little critical comment.

Every woman who attended the Women's Retreat with Domar (as with the vast majority of regular monthly RESOLVE meetings) was white, and most, judging from their dress and speech, were middle or upper-middle class. Yet RESOLVE meetings generally were silent on the issues of class and race privilege built into the use of ART. I often expected the topics of class and race to emerge in discussions about health insurance coverage, of which there were many, but what I observed instead would be more accurately described as an insiders' commiseration about experiences and expectations that are class- and race-specific.

In general, discussion participants proactively sought medical care for their infertility, had access to good medical care, and were willing to find ways to finance high-tech reproduction. They also tended to feel strongly that infertility treatments should be covered by insurance. However, most of my interviewees, with the notable exception of one of the RESOLVE copresidents, did not couch their opinions about insurance coverage in terms of what would be fair for society.[31] They tended to talk about the financial hardship that ART had presented to them personally and about the trade-offs they felt they had to make to afford treatments, including forgoing new houses or vacations to pay for another cycle of IVF (as discussed in chapter 3). In other words, they experienced the hardship—as anyone would—through the lens of their socioeconomic status. The crisis of infertility made them more aware of what they were giving up in relation to their peers. And how they described the crisis made it more evident to me who their peers actually were—middle- and upper-middle-class professionals. Among those who did have insurance coverage, at least one, a former RESOLVE leader, questioned her motives for trying IVF when the insurance company was paying for it.

So what compelled these people, with or without insurance, to try ART and in some cases to keep trying it? What about this group's class- or race-specific expectations made these people vulnerable? Based on economist Juliet Schor's observations about American society, I believe that "belonging to a particular social class now entails consuming a requisite set of goods and services."[32] In this case, the requisite set of goods and services was ART. Schor, drawing on Pierre Bourdieu's *Distinction: A Social Critique of the Judgment of Taste* (1984), makes the point that "Bourdieu argues that not only economic class but also what he calls 'cultural capital' affect consumption patterns. In his view, people acquire cultural capital through family socialization and educational background, and this cultural capital shapes their tastes and preferences. Taste becomes an expression of class position, as do the consumer choices associated with it."[33] I think viewing the use of ART as a consumer choice that expresses the "tastes"—or at least the values and expectations—of a particular social class is a reasonable way to interpret RESOLVE. Members of this group, generally speaking, expected unfettered access to high-quality medical services. They valued their ability to master problems. They were accustomed to the use of technology. All of these values and expectations likely reinforced their attraction to ART.

Consuming ART makes sense in light of certain class-specific expectations about the "life course," a term used by John Meyer to describe the standardized scripts or institutional recipes on which individuals draw as they work out their identities over time.[34] From Meyer's perspective, class-specific scripts structure everyone's expectations and self-definitions. For the relatively narrow population that tends to use ART in American society, that script seems to call for higher education, a professional credential or career, and childbearing as a culminating midlife project.

As helpful as it is to consider the role of class and race in the use of ART, these factors may still not fully explain why a preference for ART sometimes turns into an obsession. There may be more to the story. Getting stuck on the treadmill of infertility cannot be wholly class- or race-specific.

The Treadmill of Infertility

Scholars have raised concerns about consumerism's impact on American culture generally and on the use of ART in particular, including the "technological imperative" that seduces many infertile couples into thousands of dollars of expense.[35] Consumerism, or, as Schor describes in *The Overworked American* (1992), the "consumption ethic," entails wastefulness, self-indulgence, artificial obsolescence, and competitiveness. Consumerism also entails the creation of needs, which, according to Schor, reverses the assumptions of neoclassical economic theory: people want what they get rather than get what they need. This creation of needs is part of the "vicious work and spend cycle" that fuels overwork in American society. She dubs this cycle the "squirrel cage of capitalism."[36] Like the "treadmill of infertility," the squirrel cage of capitalism is difficult to exit, because, as Roger Rosenblatt explains in *Consuming Desires: Consumption, Culture, and the Pursuit of Happiness* (1999), "relentless yearning" always follows on the heels of "relentless getting and spending."[37] Much of this analysis applies to the phenomenon of ART.

Based on what I observed at RESOLVE meetings, the treadmill of infertility does not necessarily involve competitiveness in the sense of a prideful, aspiring "keeping up with the Joneses." A strong desire to avoid lifelong regret fueled a certain kind of competitiveness, but it was more in the sense of, "How can I *not* try this treatment if someone I know is trying it for the same problem?"[38] The treadmill of infertility also does not necessarily involve commodification, the objectification of the process and products of reproduction, although that may be an unintended consequence of ART. I think people remain on the treadmill because of the utility of ART—the needs it serves (including but not limited to the physical problem of infertility) and the needs it helps to create—which fits well with the dynamics of consumerism.

As one RESOLVE leader said, "Some people need to do one IVF, others need to do ten or more before they feel done. You can't rush the grieving process."[39] I found this statement astounding because it leads to the question of what needs IVF is serving here. She proposes that undergoing treatment plays a significant role in the grieving process of coming to terms with one's infertility. Her statement offers no expectation that treatment will work to produce a viable pregnancy. But the utility of treatment is not limited to that goal. Along similar lines, I heard discussion leaders on a few occasions suggest that going through lower-tech procedures could be useful psychologically even if there was little chance of achieving pregnancy: at least people would feel as though they were doing something. Another justification was that lower-tech treatment often helps people facing infertility gain a comfort level with high-tech treatments. Indeed, one discussion participant expressed the difficulties he and his wife had encountered in going straight to the "Star Wars stuff" without the warm-up of lower-tech treatment.

Moving forward in the grieving process, creating a feeling of doing something beneficial, gaining a comfort level with the increasing levels of intervention and medicalization—all these outcomes derive from the utility of simply consuming ART, even without the tangible benefit of a viable pregnancy. And that is what consumerism is all about. As Rosenblatt remarks, "Nothing seems to cultivate the self as does consumption."[40] Trying ART feels empowering. It meets a very basic need in terms of combating the sense of personal failure that infertility seems to cause, but it also helps to create needs that did not previously exist. Who could have imagined, even thirty years ago, that someone would need to do ten or more cycles of IVF before coming to terms with infertility?

The irony of the treadmill metaphor is that one is stationary on a treadmill; there is only the illusion of forward progress. Yet as chapter 5 will explore, this does not mean that one is not strengthened and changed by the experience. The question for this chapter is who really benefits from all the time and money spent on ART, especially when patients find themselves doing multiple trials with diminishing chances of achieving pregnancy. Can we say that people who use ART are making free—meaning uncoerced and consciously examined—choices to do so? Moreover, even if some voices within RESOLVE questioned the treadmill of ART—and a degree of ambivalence clearly existed about exhaustive efforts to achieve pregnancy—did they make a convincing case about when and how to step off the treadmill of infertility treatments?

Moral Agency, Human Flourishing, and the Common Good

Moral Agency

This chapter has discussed some of the ways that the larger social context may affect the use of ART, but members of RESOLVE rarely acknowledged or examined this context. Key to understanding why this larger context goes unnoticed and unchallenged is the ethos of moral neutrality within RESOLVE discussions. At the heart of my analysis lies an overarching interest in the question of moral agency. I am concerned with whether people are making choices unduly compromised by external forces. Beyond that, I am concerned that people recognize their power to shape the social contexts in which we all act.

"Moral agency" describes the nature of our actions as autonomous beings who are conscious of and make free choices based on their interests and values but who never entirely transcend their historical and social location. This understanding of moral agency rests on an idea of social selfhood: human beings are not Kantian agents with a narrow understanding of freedom and free choices abstracted from their social contexts (the liberal fallacy). We are both dependents and caregivers, in Kittay's language, and we are fellow citizens in community with each other, in the language of H. Richard Niebuhr, whose actions can cause harm to the community even if they do not harm individual members. Yet despite our socially shaped existence, we do not mindlessly live out social structures (the structuralist fallacy). Moments of choice and freedom exist in which individuals exert their individuality, creativity, and dignity and push back against or depart from determining social conditions. The extremes of social determinism and pure volunteerism bracket a space in which it is possible to honor the life plans and desires of individuals while reflecting critically on the ends toward which individuals strive and the social structures in which we live.

Exercising this moral agency—perhaps better termed "reflective and responsive self-determination," to build on Niebuhr's ideas—requires an awareness of a larger social context. Merely having this awareness does not enable one to transcend one's social context, to make decisions utterly unaffected by cultural norms and expectations. But without any reflection on the larger social context, one's "free" choices are more vulnerable to external forces, as Cahill expresses when she says that when autonomy is unchallenged as the supreme value in human action, a vacuum is created into which can flow the "still strong forces of patriarchy and market economics" as well as our naive faith in technology.[41] Free choices, like the decision to delay childbearing, to use ART, to be an egg donor, and so forth, need to be examined with an awareness of social structures, including those that have historically worked to women's disadvantage.

However, my ability to assess whether other people have an "awareness of a larger social context" is subjective, which raises the challenge posed by Charles Kurzman, a sociologist who writes about biases inherent in ethnographic research.[42] Kurzman argues that the "social distance" between researcher and subjects influences how the subjects are judged. He explains the two pairs of dichotomous metatheoretical values governing researchers' assessments of their subjects. The first pair includes "respect for subjects" versus "social silencing," while the second pair includes "social determinism" versus "volunteerism." As the labels suggest, the first pair describes researchers' assessments of their subjects' knowledge or self-awareness: researchers either listen to and respect the subjects' analysis of their situation (respect for subjects) or believe that "social forces systematically prevented the subjects from properly understanding their own situation" (social silencing). The second pair speaks to researchers' assessments of the subjects' behavior, which is either held to be caused by broad social forces (social determinism) or transcends determining social forces (volunteerism).

According to Kurzman, "Both of these dichotomies operated on a continuum of social distance from our subjects: When we felt closer to them, we were more likely to respect their analyses and to grant them free will. When we felt distanced, we saw their analyses as systematically deluded and their behavior as socially determined."[43] His point about social distance between researcher and researched serves as an important reminder that ethnographic researchers, their biases, and their social location constitute a part of the research itself. Acknowledging that fact, however, does not delegitimate the project of ethnographic research or settle the question of moral agency. There is no purely objective perspective from which to judge, only a commitment to be both empathetic and analytical.

In assessing my research subjects' level of awareness of the social context in which they decide and act, I have raised concerns about the social scripts about childbearing and other life choices that are presented to women, the scripts presented to the professional classes about the timing of childbearing and career, and the scripts presented to all Americans about the therapeutic value of consumption.[44] If we begin with the premise that all "free" acts are embedded in a social context and that no one completely disengages from the available social scripts, perhaps the deeper normative agenda of this chapter is to consider the meaning of freedom more broadly and to challenge existing scripts associated with the use of ART. If RESOLVE is something of a stage—or at least an institution that embodies many important values about how one is supposed to negotiate infertility—then we need to attend more closely to its espoused ethos of neutrality.

"True" agency to at least some degree requires considering the "final ends" of ART and engaging in some "reflective and responsive" moral reasoning rather than living out a script. I do not mean to imply that everyone needs a polished argument about why they are using ART before trying it, only that they can avoid inadvertently becoming stuck on the treadmill of infertility and that they ought to have more support from RESOLVE in questioning this unhealthy script.

The Purpose and Significance of Pursuing Treatment

In general, participants in RESOLVE discussions were very reluctant to impose moral judgments on each other about any aspect of "resolving" infertility. What mattered was the worthy goal of building a family. How that goal was achieved was a matter of personal choice based on individual values and what was feasible medically, financially, and legally. The benefits of this open-minded approach were many: respect for different types of family forms, respect for the social bonds and voluntary commitments that make a family, and compassion for suffering. But the limitations were also clear: the emphasis on private freedom of choice makes it difficult to have a collective discussion about the larger purpose and value of pursuing treatment. It also makes it difficult to question the goal of building a family and difficult to abandon that goal altogether.

A few voices within RESOLVE tried to have a collective discussion about the larger purpose and value of pursuing treatment. Usually they were people who had chosen to be child-free—the minority in RESOLVE—and had discovered that what ultimately mattered most to them was not building a family but rather saving the self and saving a marriage from being destroyed by infertility. These voices asked when enough was enough, raised the issue of stopping treatment, and questioned external pressures to continue treatment or adopt. However, even these voices had difficulty articulating their point because the language of neutrality gave them so little to say that made sense. Even when the norm of neutrality could be shown to be inaccurate—after all, RESOLVE firmly believes that family building is a good—no familiar vocabulary existed for asserting and defending other important values, such as the idea that human flourishing depends on more than the freedom to pursue unlimited treatment or to pursue any conceivable goal. The reflexive language of neutrality had little room for substantive considerations of what constitutes a "good" life, choice, relationship, or person. Nor did this language have the capacity to interpret the significance of the broader context and the implications of personal choices.

In this arena, the tools and language of ethical analysis could contribute a great deal to the conversation. At their best, traditions in philosophical and religious ethics can be sources of insight and clarification, even empowerment. Ethics can provide a way of thinking through the meaning and significance of choices. And at the very least, it can raise questions that might not otherwise get raised.

As an example, I will again return to the physician who addressed the RESOLVE group about using the Internet to gather information about the latest scientific studies and newest treatment options. In addition to circumscribing his area of expertise—he could help participants only with obtaining medical information—he reinforced the idea that one's "values" in decision making were "personal" and private. He claimed not to be able to offer any substantive advice about why any one course of action would be better than another: he was there solely to convey neutral information. "I can't make these decisions for you. This is such personal stuff. I can only educate you about the choices."[45]

Yet before the evening ended, he offered at least one piece of advice. To the women in the group, he said, "If you're over thirty-eight, the most cost-effective plan is to use donor eggs."[46] No one seemed to react negatively to this advice, at least overtly, perhaps because most people assume that finding what is most "cost-effective" is a wise and utterly natural step in the decision-making process. As I listened, however, I wondered about the other steps in the decision-making process that were not receiving attention and the implicit normative judgment that goes unnamed when one prioritizes cost-effectiveness.[47]

This comment, which came from one physician and which remained unchallenged by the group, is significant for what it represents about late capitalist American culture: we have forgotten how to talk about ends but are well equipped with a vocabulary for talking about means. In other words, we know how to calculate or navigate our way from point A to point B but are less inclined and less able to reflect on the value or meaning of point B, especially when we are in the company of others pursuing that same end. I join a long line of scholars and cultural critics who have made this criticism, beginning with Max Weber's predictions in the early twentieth century about the "iron cage" of capitalism and developing the idea that the spread of instrumental or strategic reason has eclipsed our ability to consider "ultimate values."[48] Weber believed that modernization meant increasing bureaucratization, secularization, and individualism. He predicted that the narrowing of rationality to means-ends calculations (instrumental reason) would hold us captive to market values whose ultimate worth we would forget how to question.

Building on Weber's insights, Jürgen Habermas argues that the political and economic systems of capitalist societies have invaded and "colonized" what he calls the "lifeworld"—the world of lived experience and meaning making, including ethical norms, religion, and culture. Habermas and those who have developed his ideas have not accepted the iron cage metaphor as the final word on advanced capitalist societies such as our own but have endeavored to find new understandings of reason that are more than instrumental, including the use of reason in dialogue with others to arrive at norms of justice. These theorists have not given up on the Enlightenment idea that such things as shared norms of justice exist and that through an intersubjective process, human beings can find them.[49]

Cahill and Martha Nussbaum—one a theological ethicist and the other a philosophical ethicist—also care deeply about recovering a use of reason as "practical" or moral rather than merely instrumental or technical. Cahill is more inspired by Habermas and critical theory, Nussbaum sees herself working more in the liberal tradition of justice theorist John Rawls, but both share the goal of trying to develop substantive norms of justice. In their willingness to describe substantive as opposed to purely procedural visions of justice, they part company from Habermas and Rawls. However, for the purposes of this discussion, such a difference can be understood at the level of an internal family dispute. At bottom, all of these theorists embrace the use of reason for deliberating questions of the right and the good—a considerably different enterprise from technical means-ends calculations. For example, they would have problems with our ability to use reason to accomplish a sophisticated scientific task such as cytoplasmic transfer, for example, without also possessing the ability to use our reason to deliberate about the moral significance of this technique, how it is used, who has access to it, and what its impact will be—including its impact on the children born through it and on society as a whole.

Because they are neo-Aristotelians, both Cahill and Nussbaum believe that human life is purposeful and aims at happiness (that is, it is eudaemonistic). Moreover, the goods that constitute happiness are real—they have "objectivity" and "stability" and can be known through human reason. According to Cahill,

> The way in which [these goods] are known is not by examining the structures of reason itself, but by inductive reflection on, and generalization from, human experiences of need, of lack or deprivation, of fulfillment and flourishing, and of social cooperation. Moral knowledge, in this view, is not read directly from experience as a sheer fact; the existence of a practice or its wide acceptance cannot as such yield a moral law. Morality requires reasonable reflection on human existence, fine discrimination of goods whose possession truly constitutes happiness, and judgments about which activities lead to those goods and which do not.[50]

When we look to experience to find out which activities lead to human flourishing and which do not, we typically look for commonalities. We generalize, despite the great variety in human existence, and thereby run the risk of "essentializing"—an oppressive move if it obliterates difference. However, both Cahill and Nussbaum argue that respect for particularity and difference does not mean that normative assessments are impossible.[51] Infinitely variable answers do not exist to the question of how a human being should live. The commonalities across human experience, even if very basic or minimal, make it possible to say that life is better than death, bodily health and integrity is better than illness and violence, and so on.

Cahill grounds her vision of human flourishing in her belief that human experience is bodily, intersubjective, and social, drawing on the ideas of Aristotle, Aquinas, and Catholic social thought. Nussbaum approaches the question of human flourishing from the perspective of developing a list of "central human functional capabilities"[52]—those basic capabilities that she believes all human beings need. She draws her ideas from Aristotle, Mill, and Kant.[53] It is certainly open to debate whether their substantive criteria are the best or only criteria we could imagine when assessing whether any given activity promotes human flourishing. The important point is that these categories expand the discussion beyond the simple "How can I achieve my goal?"

Both Cahill and Nussbaum believe that ethics needs continually to ask, "What does human flourishing look like, and on what does it depend?" and "How well does this activity / object / condition promote human flourishing?" Without a conception of human flourishing, we have nothing to say to the deeply relativistic claims of cost-benefit analysis, for example, which tends to flatten out the meaning of a "good" choice to a merely efficient one. We have no way of sorting through all the options for resolving infertility and lack a clear means of resisting the "treadmill of infertility"—the seduction to try more and more treatments until something works. We also have no motivation and no language to consider the impact of using a donor egg on the created child or the parents' relationship, or what it means to be an older parent, or how the social practice of using ART impacts the common good generally and the well-being of women in particular. All of these factors are defined at the outset as irrelevant because they do not count as either literal costs or benefits (for example, how much money will be spent on the procedure and whether the procedure will result in the birth of the desired baby).

To discuss the final ends of ART is not to inquire necessarily about the most effective, least expensive procedure or the one with the highest "take-home baby rate." It is to discuss whether ART promotes human flourishing and in so doing to discuss what we mean by human flourishing. It is to put aside the claim to neutrality, that all choices are equally good, and to discern which choices are better and why.

Private Choices and Their Broader Implications

Were it possible to extrapolate how participants in the RESOLVE discussions might respond to my suggestion to consider the final ends of ART, they would likely object to being asked to do something that the "fertile world" is free not to do: reflect consciously on the reasons for having children and becoming parents. The unfairness of infertility would be compounded by the unfairness of an expectation to justify choices that seem entirely natural. Many people experience the inability to reproduce as a painful exclusion from one of life's most basic processes. Moreover, one could easily argue, to be a parent to a child is surely conducive to human flourishing—from the point of view of the child who benefits from his or her parent's love and care; from the point of view of society, which will eventually benefit from parental investment in the child; and from the point of view of the parent. Thus, if the ability exists to assist people to reproduce, why not use it?

One reason it is difficult to consider this question in any depth, as I have suggested, is the pervasive belief that choices of this kind are private. The decision to use ART is perceived to affect only—or most directly and mean-ingfully—the decision makers themselves. The users of ART bear the expense, undergo the health risks, and must feel comfortable that the decision comports with their values. This private sphere of decision making is perceived to be fairly self-contained and well protected by procreative liberty, and the only way to open it up to challenge or discussion is to demonstrate tangible harm to others. Short of any tangible harm—and shockingly little data has been gathered regarding the long-term health of children born through ART procedures—people should be free to procreate however they can, or so the argument goes.[54]

However, it is helpful to recognize that this view of procreative liberty has a history and that voices and traditions within ethics have always challenged this perspective. A host of scholars—feminists, communitarians, social justice theorists, Christian ethicists, and many others—have criticized the argument for "presumptive procreative liberty"[55] on the grounds that it is deeply unrealis-tic, takes for granted the communal structures that must be in place for any exercise of individual liberty, promotes a contractual and commodified view of reproduction and children, and unfairly distributes access to reproductive assistance.[56] Yet the assumptions of unlimited procreative liberty find wide expression in public argumentation in our society through "rights talk,"[57] which accentuates the perception that people have the "right to be let alone" provided they are not harming others, and through important court decisions that tend to draw on this narrow version of individual liberty.[58]

John Robertson embraces this view of procreative liberty and the background assumptions about private and public on which it rests.[59] Robertson dispenses with concerns about harm to children by embracing Derek Parfit's circular argument that it is always better to have been born, regardless of the circumstances (diminished or enhanced); thus, there is no logical way to argue "wrongful life." He also defends the idea that reproductive decisions are private using the Supreme Court's reasoning: such decisions are acts of personal definition, central to personal identity as expressions of individuals' beliefs about the meaning of life.[60]

RESOLVE's national office has picked up this language in its publications advocating mandatory health insurance coverage, including Supreme Court language from a 1998 ruling that defines reproduction as "major life activity."[61] RESOLVE argues that the right to procreate is a "fundamental human right" and that society therefore has a moral obligation to provide access to health services for treatment of infertility. The language of rights and entitlement runs through local RESOLVE discussions as well, especially around the issue of health insurance coverage, although a few women believed that insurance coverage generally served the interests of physicians and clinics more than patients.

Upon reflection, it is hard to maintain that the "private" decision to use ART does not impact others. Susan Wolf, for example, argues that reproductive decisions are never only about the decision makers but always have implications for yet-to-be-born persons and for society generally.[62] Speaking from her personal experience with IVF treatments and from her perspective as a feminist, she believes that acceding to everything "aspiring parents" desire invites exploitation and that we need instead a "shared culture of parentalism" with an accompanying sense of duty to future children.

Where is the line between private choices and harm to others or between individual freedom and the common good? These distinctions are not easily drawn, especially in an area such as assisted reproduction, which always involves decision making on behalf of potential children. It is useful, however, to recognize that the belief that all ethical decision making is private is a metaethical commitment whose validity is open to debate.

RESOLVE members generally lacked the vocabulary to question the category of private choice as well as the goal of cost-effectiveness and the means-ends reasoning that accompanies it. RESOLVE members also had difficulty resisting the role of informed consumer, which was a self-conception blatantly reinforced by clinic representatives and physicians. Moreover, the consumer-ist orientation of RESOLVE members received powerful reinforcement from the ideology of choice and rhetoric of procreative liberty. These conceptual categories made sense to this group even as people admitted to having no idea how to navigate all the available options for treating infertility.

An ideology of choice ultimately convinces people that they are making private, self-determining choices when precisely the lack of critical reflection about and responsiveness to a larger social context undermines the possibility that self-determining choices will, in fact, be actualized. We need to fill up the vacuum left by the language of choice: only collective critical discussion can ensure that decisions do not serve harmful ends.

Critique of RESOLVE

Institutions Are Moral

Although the common understanding was that RESOLVE meetings func-tioned as a forum, which suggests an empty or open space where people gather to discuss, the meetings were part of a centralized organization with deep moral commitments to its members and to educating the public generally about infertility. These commitments entailed unconditional support and ac-ceptance of people in crisis and defending the good of family life.

In *The Good Society* (1991), Robert Bellah and his coauthors explain that institutions "mediate the relations between self and world," including "our ultimate moral (and religious) commitments."[63] They embody "a set of mutual expectations" and have "built-in ideas about how to act and implicit notions of right and wrong."[64] In short, as the *Good Society* authors contend, we live through institutions, although our radical individualism tends to obscure that reality. People came to RESOLVE meetings believing, as Bellah suggests most Americans believe, "that institutions are there to serve the private ends of individuals."[65] In this case, the end was having a baby. But whether or not they recognized it, RESOLVE members were also participating in the mediation of moral and religious understandings—in the development of values about in-fertility, ART, adoption, living without children, marriage, family, the future, hope, and many other things.

Behind my observations lies a larger debate about the nature of institutions in a pluralistic society. It is very difficult in contemporary American society to engage in the kind of collective, civil debate that some scholars have argued is the hallmark of democracy. Individuals think of themselves as "interest max-imizers" and judge their institutions according to how effectively they serve diverse, privately determined ends. Indeed, Bellah and many others fear that

Americans will become or have already become accustomed to living in an "administered society" marked by passivity before large, corporate interests.[66]

Alternatively, institutions could be viewed as sites of broader social criticism or interest formulation.[67] To recognize that institutions are inherently moral is to begin to move beyond viewing them as purely instrumental or somehow separate from the values and commitments that we confer on them. If it is true that we live through institutions, then individuals' presence and participation in an organization such as RESOLVE actively shape that institution. It represents not an empty, neutral space but a live performance.

As new members join RESOLVE and rise to its leadership positions, they have a continuing obligation to reflect on the organization's moral commitments and to make that reflection an explicit part of the activities at the local and national levels. The mission of supporting the infertile is undertaken in good faith, I believe, but understanding what constitutes "support" requires reflection on the ends of ART and responsiveness to the larger context in which it is being used.

Ambiguous Location and Loyalties

Contrary to its self-description as an "oasis of clear guidance with no strings attached,"[68] RESOLVE is multiply indebted and ambiguously located between its vulnerable membership and an infertility industry that seeks to capture the market of infertile patients. RESOLVE bears a quite literal debt to the financial sponsorship of pharmaceutical companies and to local fertility clinics and physicians. For example, one drug company, Serono, was a major benefactor of RESOLVE's annual National Infertility Awareness Week. Serono's literature was available to RESOLVE members at local meetings, and the company's advertisements supported the newsletters. Each monthly RESOLVE meeting also had financial sponsors, a list of which was displayed on a board at the front of the room where people met. Sponsors were usually area clinics, especially if they were responsible for the formal presentation part of the meeting (such as the meeting about egg donors), and pharmaceutical companies.

Thus, although RESOLVE is a nonprofit organization, it is closely tied to for-profit companies and clinics. These ties with industry obviously keep the organization running, including enabling it to sustain its lobbying efforts. These ties also provide the benefit of greater access to cutting-edge information, which infertility patients eagerly seek. However, RESOLVE's relationship with industry also creates a potentially very serious conflict of interest. RESOLVE as an organization must constantly balance its stated advocacy for its members against the for-profit agendas of its financial sponsors. RESOLVE's loyalty to doctors and clinics and drug companies does not necessarily always conflict with its loyalty to RESOLVE members, but this situation makes it more difficult to assess whose interests are being served and to challenge the "treadmill of infertility."

Serving the Interests of the Infertile?

The bioethics community evidences growing concerns about the lack of scientific data on the long-term effects of the drugs used in ART procedures on both women and the children conceived through ART. Such studies apparently are difficult to fund.[69] Some people have even suggested that ART may be the next diethylstilbestrol (DES).[70] Some preliminary data link ART with ovarian cancer, and one study suggests that children born through ART are at increased risk for birth defects.[71] That no data as yet confirm or allay concerns about the health risks of ART is less significant, I think, than RESOLVE's silence on the issue of safety.

As a self-described advocate for the infertile, RESOLVE should be taking a stronger stand on the safety of ART. It cannot consistently claim to support the interests of the infertile and not also do what it can to protect the health and safety of the women who use ART and the children born through it. RESOLVE could advocate funding for more studies or take a more active role in educating its membership about health risks. At the very least, it could do more to make sure people accurately understand their chances for successful conception. I was surprised to see on RESOLVE's national Web site the claim that "Roughly ⅔ of couples who seek medical intervention are able to give birth. The most important thing you can do is to be an informed consumer."[72] Since only a little more than a quarter of women using ART have babies, I found ⅔ misleading. Without an accompanying explanation of what is meant by "medical intervention," which could include a wide range of low- and high-tech treatments, it would be easy for a first-time visitor to the site to come away with a very optimistic impression of her chances for success, especially if she assumed that medical intervention meant ART. Although there is nothing wrong with conveying a hopeful outlook, RESOLVE owes infertile patients accurate and detailed information.

In addition to taking a stronger stand on safety issues and responsible patient education, I believe RESOLVE should be more cautious in endorsing, either explicitly or implicitly, a philosophy of unlimited procreative liberty. The moral justification for egg freezing or a career pill or other hypothetical technologies on the horizon for expanding reproductive choice depends on the argument for unlimited procreative liberty, not on the argument that infertility is an illness that should be treated like other illnesses. In blurring the line between compassionate treatment for an illness and elective procedure to expand choice, RESOLVE risks delegitimating its core mission (support for the infertile) and endorsing some potentially harmful techniques.

RESOLVE's acceptance of material support from those with a vested financial interest in maintaining the treadmill of infertility, coupled with the group's silence on issues of health risks related to ART, calls seriously into question whether advancing the interests of people experiencing infertility is RESOLVE's true primary objective. RESOLVE needs to pay greater attention to the question of whose interests are really being served by its advocacy.

The President's Council on Bioethics

In 2004, the President's Council on Bioethics issued a report, *Reproduction and Responsibility: The Regulation of New Biotechnologies*, that offers a comprehensive examination of the use of ART in the United States.[73] The report culminates in a set of policy recommendations to the president, mostly calling for greater regulation of the infertility industry. RESOLVE's official interactions with the council, then chaired by Leon Kass, provide a unique opportunity to view RESOLVE's advocacy in action and to debate the organization's priorities. RESOLVE successfully lobbied the council to modify some of the report's final recommendations.

As part of the process of gathering information about assisted reproduction and its regulation in the United States, the President's Council on Bioethics asked officials from the United Kingdom's Human Fertilisation and Embryology Authority (HFEA) to testify about how assisted reproduction is regulated in that country.[74] One revealing point of comparison is the way the two countries handle the number of embryos that can be transferred back to a woman's uterus during a single cycle of IVF. According to the chair of HFEA, British policy limits transfer to no more than two embryos at a time.

In the United States, however, no regulations govern how many embryos may be transferred back to a woman's uterus at one time. Consequently, the matter remains subject solely to the patient's desire and the doctor's discretion, provided there is informed consent on the part of the patient. Because there is the perception that transferring more embryos increases the chances that one will implant and grow into a full-term fetus and because lack of insurance coverage for ART often exerts financial pressure on patients to succeed on the first cycle of IVF, many American patients are understandably motivated to transfer three or more embryos. In fact, according to the Centers for Disease Control's 2001 ART Report, 32 percent of ART cycles using never-frozen, nondonor eggs transferred four or more embryos. Unfortunately, this practice has resulted in a marked increase in multiple births in the United States. Multiple-gestation pregnancies carry significant health risks for mothers and babies, including increased risk of prematurity and increased infant mortality. An overall increase in the U.S. infant mortality rate in 2002—the first such increase in forty years—was attributed, in part, to increased fertility treatments that have led to a higher rate of multiple births.[75]

Given the well-documented consequences of multiple embryo transfer, the United Kingdom's policy of limiting the number of embryos that can be transferred looks like a reasonable regulation. It is also fairly typical of HFEA's general approach to regulating assisted reproduction: it does not thwart progress or unduly restrict patient freedom but protects the health of all parties involved and affirms the public's confidence in the safety of these procedures. HFEA also solicits public input and discussion and formulates public policy out of this shared vision of a healthful and moral medical practice. By contrast, the laissez-faire approach in the United States, with informed consent as the only ethical requirement for how many embryos to transfer, may be the clearest illustration yet of the American ideology of choice operating in a vacuum of other moral concerns.

Moved by the United Kingdom's example and by all of its fact-finding, the President's Council has tried to bring the concern about the health of the children born through ART procedures to the forefront of public awareness. The report recommends greater protection for the consumers of ART—that is, women. Many people may not realize that the council's recommendations encountered some significant opposition from RESOLVE.

For example, the council called for more long-term studies of the physical and psychological health of children born through ART. Since health problems might not make themselves evident until later in life, it seems reasonable to follow the outcomes of these technologies by studying the children born from them over a period of many years. However, RESOLVE objected to this recommendation in its earliest formulation, citing concerns about invasion of patient privacy and an increased stigma that would result from "government surveillance." In response to this criticism, the council revised its language in the final version of its report to underscore that all participation in long-term studies would be entirely voluntary. This emphasis on voluntary participation seemed to appease RESOLVE, although I remain puzzled that a recommendation to study the long-term safety of ART would have met with strong resistance from an organization that purports to represent the interests of the infertile. The interests of the infertile presumably are large enough to include the health of the children they may someday parent.

Another example was the council's recommendation to improve the existing Fertility Clinic Success Rate and Certification Act of 1992 by adding some new requirements, including mandating that the costs of treatment be reported and that success rates be reported according to individual patient numbers rather than individual cycles of IVF. It is somewhat misleading to look only at success rates according to numbers of cycles performed because those rates do not tell you how many cycles any given patient attempted before becoming pregnant. Reporting success rates by patient numbers would more accurately represent the chances for success. Yet both of these recommendations encountered fierce opposition from RESOLVE. RESOLVE's board of directors and director of government affairs complained that the 1992 law already reported plenty of data and in fact was thereby restricting patient freedom of choice and access to services. The RESOLVE officials claimed that the current reporting system "had in some cases had the effect of hurting patients who were denied treatment because their lowered chance of having a baby dissuaded clinics from treating them and risking their statistics."[76] And objecting to "government surveillance of the cost of fertility treatment," RESOLVE insisted that consumers were capable of figuring out the costs of treatment for themselves and that a pooled database of information "did not serve their interests at all."[77]

Again, I remained baffled about why RESOLVE would oppose making more information available to consumers until I looked more critically at the group's reasons: RESOLVE opposes anything that inhibits consumer choice, even (ironically) efforts at consumer protection. Their goal is less "Let the buyer beware" and more "Let us not restrict any of the options of our educated buyers." Is this advocacy for the infertile?

These examples suggest that RESOLVE's precarious balance between truly serving patients' interests and serving as an apologist for the multibillion-dollar infertility industry is tipping in favor of the infertility industry and the consumption it promotes. What complicates this appraisal is the compassionate support I observed on the local level in one RESOLVE chapter. I return to the ethos of neutrality because I believe that herein lies the organization's greatest vulnerability.

Protection from Stigma, Avoidance of Ethics

People at RESOLVE meetings generally avoided addressing difficult ethical issues and were suspicious of normative discourse. Some of this suspicion may have been well founded: academic treatments of ART often try to speak for the infertile without listening to their points of view and without taking into account their experiences. Religious leaders are often similarly presumptuous. Yet the avoidance of ethics seemed more closely tied to an avoidance of stigma and judgment, especially religiously based judgments. The people I encountered in both interviews and group discussions generally perceived religious traditions (although most people usually meant Christianity) as regarding the use of ART as wrong.

Whatever stigma remains attached to infertility or the use of ART, RESOLVE meetings provided people with a safe space in which they found protection from hurtful comments and moralizing. In light of the reality of such comments, RESOLVE's commitment to being nonjudgmental, supportive, and compassionate is understandable and laudable. However, the general exclusion or avoidance of ethical discourse limited the scope of discussion topics at RESOLVE meetings. This truncation of the discussion did a disservice to the people who could have most benefited from this kind of sustained ethical reflection.

RESOLVE's general ethos of neutrality both serves as a tool to protect members from stigma and results from an uncritical acceptance of the ideology of choice. This mechanism may not deliver the protection it intends but in fact may make members more vulnerable to an uncritical acceptance of reproductive medicine's promises. Moreover, given RESOLVE's ambiguous institutional location, its claims to neutrality are unconvincing. If the group divested itself of its indebtedness to the infertility industry, RESOLVE would be well situated to have a substantive moral conversation about ART that does not stigmatize or hurt the discussion participants but that could still raise important, critical questions about the use of ART. It could support, if it chose, a richer public discussion with neither "basement people" nor "balcony people" but honest, critical, and compassionate conversation among the people most in need of such a conversation.

If RESOLVE looked elsewhere for financial sponsorship, especially at the national level, it would be freer to take a stand against the overconsumption of ART, for example. In addition, on the local level, I think it is entirely possible to maintain a supportive environment while raising critical questions. One discussion leader in particular was exceptionally adept at doing so. One of the few child-free spokespeople, she always kept sight of the larger goal of getting one's life back. Because RESOLVE is always changing and growing with the people who join and leave it, these people can shape what the organization becomes. The interpretation of what advocacy and support for the infertile should look like remains an open question worthy of RESOLVE's further attention.

Conclusion: Fostering Critical Thinking

Ethical theory is useful for expanding the dialogue of RESOLVE discussions, a dialogue that is already deeply moral in its content. I have focused primarily on an important part of the group's ethos: the value of nonjudgmental support and the priority of freedom of choice. The emphasis on moral neutrality about private choices impeded awareness of a larger context in which decisions about infertility take place. The idea that all views are equally valid as long as they work toward resolving infertility also impeded critical discussion.

Although RESOLVE was not neutral about many important moral questions, the espoused ethos of neutrality impoverished the moral vocabulary available for challenging consumerist individualism and gendered expectations about childbearing. Without the vocabulary of ethics, which fosters critical thinking about human flourishing and issues of social justice, RESOLVE members tended not to make connections between individual experience and larger social context. In making these claims, I am more critical of leaders, physicians, and clinic representatives than of participants, who often remained silent. Yet this silence was significant. It cannot but affect their ability to exercise critical and responsive self-determination and to believe they have some power to participate in shaping and improving society's structures.

Ethicists' theoretical contributions are helpful for situating RESOLVE discussions in a wider context and for moving the focus of analysis beyond individual choices and preferences to include a consideration of social-structural issues. However, it is perhaps unfair or at least unrealistic to expect people in the midst of a major life crisis to be attentive to or even conscious of this wider context. What may be more realistic is to reformulate Cahill's concern about the lack of critical discussion about the "final values or ends for which reproductive clients act" as a question: In what ways do RESOLVE's monthly meetings consider the "final ends" of ART? In this realm, listening to the voices of the infertile brought some unexpected insights.

In the next chapter, I will develop more fully the lessons from experience that are crucial for ethics to hear, including the significance of stories of transformation that people told as they emerged from the infertility experience. I will also discuss specific emergent group norms relating to children, parenting, and families. I consider the engagement to be two-way, including what ethics could offer and what it could stand to learn. Ethicists may lack the bodily knowledge that so profoundly affects perspective.

FIVE

Lessons from Experience

Meaning Making and the Limits of
Assisted Reproductive Technologies

In the Presence of Suffering

Making the transition from theory to lived reality is a profound experience. It is one thing to theorize about the factors that influence an individual's decision to use ART or even to criticize that decision. It is quite another to sit with the anguish of people who, month after month, find the strength to cope with their disappointment and navigate the options on the path to resolving infertility. While I still believe contextual factors played an enormous role in individual decision making about assisted reproductive technologies (ART), I would not go so far as to say these forces "governed" decision making. Listening to the voices of users of ART forced me to recognize the dignified expressions of agency that emerged despite external pressures.

In addition to demonstrating a good deal of integrity in the choices they made, the people I observed seemed to undergo a transformation in the process of "resolving" their infertility. What ethicists would miss if they chose not to listen would be the meaning making that took place on the ground. People confronted insurmountable limits that required them to reevaluate typical American myths of control and choice, created theodicies to explain their suffering, and came away from the experience forced to reflect on ideas that many other people can avoid or at least postpone—"What does it matter where my child comes from?" "What does it mean that my life is not turning out the way I thought it would?"

A perceived loss of control—over one's body, one's future, one's life—seems to be a central and defining experience for many people who face infertility. While it is tempting to interpret this theme of control as evidence that users of ART had narrow, class-specific expectations that their lives would unfold according to a predictable timeline that included education, career, and children, such an interpretation, left to stand alone, would miss the humanity in this story. Infertility profoundly challenges people's sense of themselves as healthy, capable, and autonomous beings. It challenges their understanding of what is fair, how the world works, and the meaning of life. Surely not all people experience infertility in this way, but by the same token, surely all people know what it is to feel disappointment of some kind. If the hope of ART is that it may restore lost control, the experience of ART—both when it succeeds and when it does not—seemed to provide the occasion to confront and interpret the meaning of limits, both physical and existential. Although it is a technology with great power, ART sometimes proved to be precisely what demonstrated the illusory nature of control.

That said, much can be learned from the contributions of participants and presenters at RESOLVE meetings who lived through the experience of infertility and came back to talk about it. Their continued participation in RESOLVE in itself signifies that the group's discussions cannot be reduced to a forum for the rhetoric of free choice. These veterans of infertility had important insights to impart to others and were deeply committed to helping people see their way to embracing a "life after infertility," or what could be called a wider generativity. They recognized the critical role of story or narrative in making sense of the "unique grief" of infertility and saw that the climax of this story is the transformation of self. People learned about the limits of ART and about human limits generally. Ethicists have much to learn from listening to these stories, rooted as they are in embodied knowledge.

Finally, ART presses us to define what we mean by the goods of the family. After hearing accounts of egg donation, adoption, parenting after infertility, and living child-free, I can say that people who experience infertility tend to give a great deal of thought to the meaning of family. Moreover, with more firsthand experience on which to draw, it would seem that their meaning making in the area of family is at least as valid as that of ethicists who raise objections to the use of ART. I conclude this chapter with a critique of ethics without losing the sense of "both / and" that lies at the heart of this book: ethical analyses need to be more nuanced, and RESOLVE needs to be more open to critical self-reflection, including challenging the "treadmill of infertility."

Confronting Limits and the Myth of Control

The Problem That ART Does Not Entirely Solve

One of the most consistent themes that emerged in the group discussions and interviews centered on the issue of control. Rare was the meeting when control—or, more precisely, lack of control accompanied by feelings of helplessness, anger, and frustration—did not surface as a topic of discussion. And when I asked individual interviewees, "How is the infertility problem different from other problems you have faced in your life?," I invariably heard that infertility is different if not unique because of the perceived loss of control.

For example, participants expressed a common sense that infertility challenges our ability to control or at least roughly to plan the timing of reproductive activity. One therapist who addressed the group articulated that she "grew up thinking reproduction was going to be a choice," only to find out that "it's beyond our control."[1] Couples often spend so long trying not to become pregnant, she noted, that they are surprised and unsettled when their bodies do not cooperate with the change in plans. She shared her experience with ART: she and her husband thought they would never try artificial insemination, but thirteen inseminations and a few attempts at in vitro fertilization (IVF) later, they finally decided to be child-free rather than to adopt. She commented, "The fertility process makes you try things that you never thought you'd consider."[2]

In addition to a body that is not working properly, many people cited thwarted plans for the future as part of the reason for feeling a loss of control. After learning that her most recent IVF cycle had not resulted in a pregnancy, one woman explained during a group discussion, "I'm so angry that we're having to go through this. I'm totally consumed by this right now." She said she never thought she would get married, but when her future husband proposed, she was thrilled and had many expectations about what married life would be like and how many children she would have. She did not anticipate infertility.[3]

Infertility treatments seemed to compound rather than alleviate the feeling of loss of control, in part because such treatments, especially ART, are invasive, exhausting, and expensive and do not work most of the time. In addition, decision making about reproduction now involves a team of authoritative experts, not just the individual couple. However, the most important reason may be that people seemed to approach infertility treatments with the expectation that hard work and financial sacrifice would eventually bring about the desired outcome, and they were tremendously disappointed when the problem of infertility did not yield to this approach. For example, a woman I interviewed told me, "The anger came I think from lack of control. I definitely am a person who likes to be in control. I was raised that way. Where other times in my life when I have had problems, there have been ways to—if I just put enough effort, if I just put enough of something into it, I'll fix it. And it couldn't be done with this."[4] I encountered many similar expressions of shock at this reversal of normal expectations that good outcomes follow inexorably from good efforts.

It is an open question whether people who choose to pursue infertility treatments tend to have a higher-than-average confidence in their abilities to master difficult life situations through intelligence, perseverance, and financial resources. One of the few times I was directly engaged as a participant in the RESOLVE meetings, a discussion leader asked if I thought it would be interesting to study whether there was a correlation between infertility and high achievement in other areas of life. She phrased it as a correlation between infertility and "not having experienced a lot of failures."[5] Although I had no ready answer to her question, my research suggests that users of ART generally are high achievers and resourceful individuals. This perception certainly was widely held. At a meeting with a panel presentation by three area therapists, one therapist commented that people going through infertility treatments often find it very "humbling," as she did: "It is hard for people who tend to be more independent and self-sufficient, and who are used to setting goals and meeting them. . . . You need to go through a whole grieving process."[6] She also said the infertility experience stirs up feelings that adults have when they are out of control or in someone else's control.

At a subsequent meeting, a different therapist explained to the group that infertility can pose special challenges if and when it reopens old issues or brings up old failures. One participant, a professional woman recently married, responded, "I understand what you're saying about infertility bringing up old failures, but the thing is, I haven't had a lot of failures in my life. I've always been able to figure out what I wanted and then work hard to get it. This is the first thing in my life that I haven't been able to succeed at no matter how hard I try or how much money I spend . . . and I am incredibly frustrated. I don't know what to do with all this frustration."[7] All of these expectations—especially the expectation that problems can be solved by hard work and if necessary financial sacrifice—derive from a characteristically American but more specifically upper-middle-class faith in humans' power to control the uncontrollable, to overcome obstacles through determination, and to exploit the benefits of sophisticated technologies when they are available. I think a general acceptance of the myth of control played a significant role in motivating the initial pursuit of infertility treatment in many instances.

After people embark on the treatment process, it is difficult to untangle whether they question the myth of control as a consequence of the infertility itself, the unpredictability of the treatment outcomes, or both. Some people expressed great appreciation for their infertility treatments, especially when pregnancy was "achieved," but most expressed a degree of ambivalence regardless of the outcome. Many success stories were punctuated by false starts and failures along the way: drugs that did not work, chemical pregnancies,[8] ectopic pregnancies, pregnancies that were well established but ended in miscarriage.

One woman who had success in using IVF with her own eggs (after suffering a miscarriage with an earlier cycle of IVF) said in an interview, "You know, between IVFs, we were only taking a month off, which was great for me because you don't have to grieve, you don't have to worry, you just get right back into it and go. As long as I was doing something, I was fine. I was in control—I thought—and I was working towards a goal. You know, every week you were going and getting monitored, so you'd have more information, and it was like textbook. Everything was going great. And, finally, different drugs, different things, the fourth time, we were able to get pregnant."[9] Implicit in her comments, perhaps, was a degree of critical self-reflection: "I was in control—I thought," she said, qualifying her enthusiasm. In retrospect, she seemed to realize the limited nature of her control over the process and how much the ritual of infertility treatments functioned largely to keep her mind off her grief.

A few people I interviewed, both inside and outside of RESOLVE, candidly expressed very negative opinions about ART, and in at least one case, the criticism was tied closely to the issue of control:

> I don't have an overall favorable view. . . . I think it presents it like it's too easy, like, "Well, you can just wait till you're forty." It's *not* that easy, and it's *not* that successful. . . . If you really start to break down the statistics, and I just did a little bit of looking into that, the statistics really aren't that successful for people who would have been in my age category. I mean, there's a chance, but it goes way down, it's like 20 or 25 percent—maybe. So I mean all these statistics are a little bit inflated. So I think it gives people a false notion that . . . you really have more control than you do. I mean, I think it gives you this idea that you can control it. You know, because here we were controlling it by *not* getting pregnant. That was easy. So, why can't then we just get pregnant? Even if there are responsible people giving responsible statistics, I think the effect of it is there is an idea that you can really control it.

When I asked what generated that idea, the woman continued, "There are a lot of success stories. Who talks about the non–success stories? You don't really hear about the people who tried and tried and it still didn't work. I think we're kind of a society that feels like we can control a lot anyway, so it plays right into what we like to think about ourselves."[10] This woman chose not to join RESOLVE, giving the reason that she was under the impression that RESOLVE members were on a "fast track" toward using ART. Although her impression was probably accurate, a few RESOLVE members whom I interviewed also sharply criticized ART, the entire infertility industry, and even the organization. Regardless of whether people seek out RESOLVE because they believe it supports and even encourages the use of ART—and many people probably do—the monthly discussions featured struggles with the limits of ART and what to do with this new experiential knowledge.

Bodily Experience and Embodied Knowledge

At one unusually small gathering in early January 2001, a woman directly asked the discussion leader, "How do you deal with the arrival of your period every month and the failure that that means?"[11] After a pause, the first and most emotional response to this question came from a man who sat beside his wife in the circle of chairs. A handsome and engaging couple, they had been relaying their difficulties with good humor. Earlier in the conversation, he had been very open about his desire to become a father, and his wife had shared her experiences with IVF. In response to this question, he expressed his sadness: "Every month, you get such high hopes," he said, gesturing high with his hands, "You say to yourself, 'This is going to be the one, this is going to be the one that works,' and you start getting all these expectations about what it's going to be like to have a baby. But then it doesn't work. We do a lot of crying. We spend a lot of time being angry."[12] As an equal partner with his wife in the pursuit of parenthood, he too mourned the lost opportunity every month.

Infertility and infertility treatments are bodily experiences, not abstractions, for the women as well as the men who go through them.[13] Even though infertility constitutes almost by definition an occasion when the body does not obey the desires of the will, bodily experience and the resultant embodied knowledge set this story apart. It would be easy to see the use of ART as just another example of human beings trying to master nature through the use of a relatively new technology. Our culture interprets most scientific breakthroughs this way, whether the story is genetically modified foods or the potential benefits of embryonic stem cells. Although some people may be uncomfortable with the continual drive to surpass "natural" limits, it is generally understood that science and medicine are indeed in the business of surpassing nature, of saving or extending life, healing illness, and creating new possibilities where none existed previously. But ART, in the end, seems not to deliver people from the limits of embodied existence so much as refocus attention on these limits and their significance.

For example, the prominence of the body for couples facing infertility challenges people who claim that the volitional aspects of human life and human relationships have triumphed over the bodily ones. In *Sex, Gender, and Christian Ethics*, Lisa Cahill argues that modern Westerners prize "intentionality and choice" and that "reproduction, in turn, has become a personal option gauged to the relational needs of sexual partners." Basing her judgment on generalizations about modern Westerners and secondhand accounts of infertility, Cahill claims that the "bodily aspects of parenthood disappear to the moral backstage, while the affective and intentional ones part the curtains to a standing ovation."[14] My work with people using or considering ART suggests, however, that rather than diminishing the moral weight of the body, the experience of infertility seems to remind people that the precious bodily aspects of parenthood cannot be taken for granted.[15]

Moreover, the disappointment in infertility is not merely a function of thwarted "intentionality and choice." When people face the limits of their bodies as well as the limits of reproductive technologies, the causes of disappointment are more complex. Part of what is lost is the understanding of the self as embodied and healthy. And in some cases, as with egg or sperm donation, surrogacy, and adoption, part of what is lost are the connections among biological, gestational, and social parenthood.

The people I observed wanted more than anything to have normal, embodied conceptions and viewed technological intervention as signifying a major adjustment. As one woman put it, "None of us expected to be here. I never expected to have to go outside my bedroom to have a child. This is a loss."[16] Describing the progression from low-tech to high-tech intervention, another woman explained that she first tried the oral drug Clomid and "thought we could at least still have sex," but then she had to "give up the dream of a romantic conception" when they moved to IVF.[17] In addition, insofar as intentional decisions to delay childbearing were perceived as contributing to fertility problems, especially for women, these choices were not usually celebrated but rather became the source of guilt or regret.

Do these remarks suggest that the myth of control was ultimately decisive? I think not, especially if one pays special attention to the voices of people on the "other side" of infertility. An irony of the infertility experience is that the body—exactly what is not acquiescing to the desires of the will—eventually schools the will to accept limits. The body provides its own knowledge and wisdom, has its own moral weight, and thus becomes more than merely an obstacle to intentionality and choice. People struggling with infertility negotiate the relationship between embodiment and volition every day. And those on the other side of infertility seem to know that the key to resolving infertility is coming to terms with what cannot be controlled.

Life after Infertility:
Meaning Making and Narratives of Transformation

The Stages of Grief

RESOLVE meetings brought together current and past sufferers of infertility. People who had "successfully resolved" their infertility came back to meetings to give presentations, to volunteer as greeters, and to participate in discussions. In fact, RESOLVE members' loyalty to the organization was striking; many boasted of being members "for life."[18] Individuals on the other side of infertility seemed to provide a great deal of hope to those currently in the throes of decision making, and a curious consistency existed in the nature of their comments, which had the benefit of hindsight and the healing effects of time. One way to interpret the consistency in these comments is that they were stylized conversion narratives. In this case, the vices of anger, bitterness, and jealousy were transformed into the virtues of acceptance, gratitude, and love through a process with predictable stages and turning points.[19]

Only toward the end of my field research did I realize how much the speakers at monthly meetings, especially the therapists, drew explicitly on Elisabeth Kübler-Ross's stages of grief in advising and counseling people.[20] At the March 2001 meeting, "Shattered Dreams: Dealing with Grief, Loss, and Anger," the discussion leader briefly described the stages of grief, including the last stage, acceptance and hope: "You will never be the same person, but your life will go on, and there will be transformation in the process."[21] The stages of grief clearly represent a sequential narrative of conversion or transformation, with predictable turning points and a hopeful trajectory. This narrative was presented to people struggling with infertility with the apparent intention of helping them heal emotionally and "resolve" their infertility.

In conjunction with an explanation of the stages of grief, an extended discussion occurred about how the infertility grieving process has its own peculiar and painful expression because the object of grief never fully existed and is more like a hope or dream or vision for oneself that included an imagined relationship with a child. For example, one woman who attended regularly was very reserved during the meetings and, unlike many of the other women, never brought her husband. She quietly spoke up during a discussion about Mother's Day/Father's Day, however. She said that her husband never spoke of his disappointment but that the two of them had the same exchange every year around Mother's Day. She would say to him, "I hate Mother's Day," and he would reply simply and kindly, "I know you hate Mother's Day."[22]

Participants acknowledged that the grief for the death of this dream and all its component parts never entirely goes away. There is no necessary endpoint to the hope for a child, and no funeral to mark the loss that infertility represents, although rituals to mark miscarriages were encouraged. As one discussion leader explained, "Childlessness gets resolved, one way or another. Infertility never does."[23] Though enigmatic, this comment suggests that childlessness is a practical problem with a few practical solutions, whereas infertility is almost akin to an existential condition. It does not get fixed as much as reintegrated into a changed understanding of the self.

Moving beyond infertility, to the "transformation" stage of grief, seemed to involve an acceptance of limits and a cessation of the desire to control. The voices of experience spoke to the difficulty of this task: "It's hard to let go of your timeline," said one RESOLVE leader sympathetically.[24] "Let go of the myths about what it's like to have a biological child," counseled another woman who had resolved her infertility through adoption.[25] Lose the attachment to the romantic notion of what it is supposed to be like to conceive a baby, she suggested, and instead focus on "having a family."

Even the pharmaceutical companies, perhaps in an effort to make themselves seem sympathetic, encouraged the acceptance of limits. The pamphlets set out at the monthly meetings included *Infertility: The Emotional Roller Coaster*, printed by Serono, a major manufacturer of infertility drugs used in IVF. The pamphlet concluded, "Here are some common feelings couples experience as they work toward resolution: acceptance of things you cannot change, realization that you can't completely control every aspect of your life, a greater ability to empathize with other people's problems, learning that 'good' things can actually come out of 'bad experiences,' life can be fulfilling even when you can't obtain all your dreams."

Something about this pamphlet is reminiscent of advertisements that counsel restraint, such as an ad for an alcoholic beverage that reads "drink responsibly" or for a credit card that cautions the consumer to "spend wisely." These companies know about the perils of alcoholism and the staggering debt that many Americans carry, yet they want people to use their product anyway. Perhaps Serono has shrewdly discerned that (1) infertility treatments can be addictive and (2) speaking the language of grief, control, and transformation taps into a powerful set of emotions. The company's advice about accepting limits thus earns the trust and loyalty of the consumer, at least for some period of time.

Moving beyond infertility ultimately involves dealing with time, the limits of the biological clock, the choices of one's past and the hopes for one's future. As people move out of the time during which they are willing to try infertility treatments—and for some people this period stretches on for years—the changes that people undergo seem to require that the whole experience be framed as a story or narrative.

Warren Reich writes that the core of suffering is "anguish over the injury or threat of injury to the self."[26] He argues that there are three phases of suffering. Phase 1 is mute suffering, the "experience of being speechless in the face of one's own suffering," where control (*nomos*) over the destiny of the self (*autos*) is threatened.[27] Phase 2 is expressive suffering, which takes the form of a story or narrative that reconfigures or reforms the deconstructive, mute experience of suffering into something new. Expressive suffering often uses metaphorical language to evoke this sense of reconfiguration and helps sufferers to work through their pain: "People in pain tell their story in the hope that they will be able to reconstruct and thus recreate their painful and dislocating past, to gain some distance from it, to put it into perspective, and thus to 'possess' their experience as a way of putting the past behind them. Second, the narrative is told in the hope that someone may affirm the sufferer in the search for a new story, a story that will account for and justify a new self that might emerge from the suffering with wholeness or identity or pride or meaning or at least with hope. What the sufferer seeks is a believable and effective narrative of life."[28] Reich contends that something is deeply significant about the tendency of suffering to be expressed as a story. The act of narrating itself, especially in communication with compassionate others, plays a crucial role in transforming the suffering. Finally, phase 3 is finding a new identity in suffering and having a voice of one's own. Here sufferers find solidarity with compassionate others and "take a stand toward the conditions" that gave rise to the suffering.

Data from my field research support Reich's account of the expressive phase of suffering and the importance of having or creating a story to make sense of the past, present, and future. The suffering caused by infertility differs from that occasioned by a sudden death, illness, or trauma in that people do not define themselves as infertile until they desire to have a child. The same person who one year is using contraception to avoid pregnancy is not infertile but rather is carrying out a desired plan for her life, which perhaps includes a desire for children—later.[29] The change in desire, in addition to a change in circumstances, creates the problem. The narratives of transformation in infertility, therefore, typically incorporated the fact that there was a prior story that had to be altered. As one RESOLVE leader suggested, "Everyone will eventually have a story, it just may not be the one you fantasized about."[30]

An emblematic narrative of transformation that incorporates a story from the past into a story about the future is the "Welcome to Holland" parable, read at two of the RESOLVE meetings I attended. In its original form, "Welcome to Holland" tells the story of parents who must adjust to having a disabled infant when they expected to give birth to and raise a "normal" child.[31] In the allegory, the reader arrives for a vacation in Holland rather than in Italy. The moral of the story is that if the traveler spends life wishing he or she had reached Italy, like everyone else and as he or she had always expected and planned, he or she will fail to appreciate all the lovely things about Holland. When the "Welcome to Holland" story was read during RESOLVE meetings, it was adapted (without acknowledging the adaptation) so that the experience of infertility substituted for the birth of the disabled infant. Holland is the metaphor for the experience of infertility, while Italy represents the fertile world. Whatever critiques could be made of this allegory or the unstated equation of infertility to parenting a disabled child (or the analogy between either experience and a European vacation!), the story was presented with the clear understanding that a transformation of self must occur. Resolving infertility (in the sense of being at peace with it) requires a sacrifice of old expectations and dreams and an embracing of a new vision for one's life.

In addition to the "Welcome to Holland" parable, I heard many personal stories of transformation from RESOLVE members who had resolved their infertility through one of the three main means (medical treatment, adoption, or deciding to remain child-free). These stories were told largely in retrospect, after a new vision for the self had been accepted, but it seems likely that individuals' narratives played a significant role in making sense of their infertility experience while it was happening. The stories provided people with tools with which to create meaning out of the past as well as to adjust to present circumstances. Sometimes but not always, these narratives drew explicitly on religious language and ideas, such as the idea of a providential design for one's life. This language and the use of allegory and metaphor suggest the degree to which meaning making was an inherent part of these group discussions.

The Path to Adoption

The all-day adoption symposium was full of examples of individual stories. One presenter at the symposium claimed, "People tell me they're *glad* they didn't become pregnant" and thus ended up adopting their particular children.[32] Another adoptive parent shared her view: "Adoption is the most spiritual experience you can have in life."[33] A discussion leader who spent the first eight years of her marriage trying infertility treatments before adopting a child explained that one of the benefits of adoption is that the parents cannot have any preconceived ideas about who children are: "You really have to discover who *they* are."[34] And at one of the first RESOLVE meetings I attended, an adoptive parent shared her conviction that a "little soul [is] out there waiting" for every person who wants to become a parent.[35]

One woman whom I chose to interview based on her comments during the adoption symposium expressed great appreciation for having been led to adoption after a painful period of soul-searching ("How could a loving God do this to somebody?") and what she described as a clinical depression after going through IVF and losing the pregnancy at nine weeks.[36] She elaborated,

> It hasn't been totally a year since we adopted the boys, but I am 100 percent earnest when I say that I would go through all the grief, all the yuck, all the expense, the time—everything—to be where we are now. And you know, I have to add that the thing that has drastically changed for me besides the fact that we now have two little boys in our house is my spiritual growth has been phenomenal, and it's this experience that brought me to that. . . . We just felt like our experience was unbelievable in that we had two gorgeous little boys that had very minor medical issues and to this day have not come up with anything more drastic, but even if they would, obviously it is something we would deal with at this point. But we just, I think, came back feeling like we didn't do this on our own. We had a lot of help from above, and that event spurred me on to do a lot of reading, a lot more soul-searching and brought me to what I believe in today. So that's why I say that I would have everything happen the same way to get where we are in our family life and where I am in my spiritual life.[37]

This woman, like many of the people interviewed, spontaneously raised the issue of faith and how much infertility had challenged her core beliefs. An essential task in meaning making is to deal with the threats to one's self-perception and worldview, or to create a theodicy that explains or justifies how "bad things can happen to good people" to make sense of the individual's crisis and the experience of infertility generally. For example, one woman wondered whether infertility "was God's way of having some kids out there in the world that don't have parents taken care of."[38]

Infertility as a Gift

In addition to the comments by people who were happy with their decision to adopt and who even expressed gratitude for the experience of infertility for leading them to adopt the particular children that are now theirs, numerous people described infertility as a gift.[39] One RESOLVE leader said, "The people that are the closest to me in Atlanta are people that I met because of going through infertility. . . . So now that I'm on the other side, yes, for me, in my life and for my faith, it was all in God's plan. It was meant for a purpose. And I'm a richer person with all these relationships. But, you know, you don't want to hear that when you're in the midst of it—'Oh, it's a gift, it's wonder-ful.' "[40] During group discussions, she repeatedly described infertility as a "life-changing event" and stated that she was not the same person that she had been. Pregnant through IVF, she expressed appreciation for the "miracle of conception" and noted that everything in her pregnancy seemed so significant.

Another interviewee explained that infertility had put a lot of pressure on her marriage, but she and her husband recently had "turned a corner" in their counseling: "I can only hope that something else would have provided that kind of opportunity for us, but I don't know. And so there was a point where I did very begrudgingly say, 'Well, I guess this infertility's been a gift, because this is what it's doing.' "[41] This woman also used the term "epiphany" to describe her experience with infertility. She had a lot of religious background and training, including the Episcopal Church's "Education for Ministry" program, but her use of religious terms was not unique.

Many people seemed to turn to religious language and imagery to describe the experience of infertility—as a "gift" or "epiphany" or "journey." This phenomenon suggests that the language of choice and control is of limited value in dealing with infertility. Infertility is not like other problems, people said time and time again, because it does not yield to the usual strategies of practical problem solving, of hard work and perseverance and purchasing the right product (in this case, expensive therapies). The use of religious imagery and language may have indicated that people felt themselves outside the realm of practical problem solving and were considering deeper existential ques-tions, including the "How should we live?" questions that are not answered by means-ends reasoning.

The experience of infertility—by which I mean not just the inability to become pregnant but the physically and emotionally exhausting treatments, the disappointments of the negative pregnancy tests, and the heartbreaking miscarriages—profoundly challenged people's faith, whether it was a faith in a loving and just God or a less explicitly theocentric faith in a just world. Many people turned to religious language because it seemed more adequate to the task of dealing with this challenge and interpreting the meaning of insur-mountable limits, including mortality.

People in the Atlanta chapter of RESOLVE may also generally have had a greater level of comfort with religious language than RESOLVE members in more secular regions of the United States. Given the limitations of my deci-sion to focus on just one RESOLVE chapter, I cannot definitively distinguish between the Atlanta chapter and other chapters. However, other scholars who study ART, including Marcia Inhorn and Gay Becker, do not share my observations. In discussing Becker's ethnography of IVF in the United States, *The Elusive Embryo: How Women and Men Approach New Reproductive Technologies* (2000), Inhorn pointedly emphasizes that "religion never surfaces" in Becker's account.[42] More specifically, Inhorn claims that "most infertile Americans engaged in the actual practice of IVF and its variants do not seem to draw upon their religions to make moral judgments [or] to help them overcome the 'meaning-threatening' aspects of infertility."[43] Instead, Inhorn believes that Becker's work clearly demonstrates that "American test-tube baby making now operates on a very secular-materialist consumer model."[44]

I disagree with this generalization based on my case study of RESOLVE of Georgia. I cannot fully account for the differences I observed, but some of the explanation may lie in regional differences within the United States, although it seems overly simplistic to attribute the entire phenomenon to easy generalizations about the South. In both group discussions and individual interviews, I witnessed a great deal of overt spiritual questioning and explanations for suffering that used religious language, despite the fact that RESOLVE is not a religiously affiliated organization. In fact, although I would agree that the secular-materialist consumer model is indeed very powerful, the members of RESOLVE I observed were not ultimately mere consumers expressing their preferences. They were also members of a meaning-making community. The fact that so many veterans of infertility—the elders of RESOLVE—attended monthly meetings to participate in this communal meaning making also supports the interpretation that RESOLVE meetings were more than seedbeds of consumption.

On the local level, RESOLVE in some ways functioned as a substitute church for its members. As I have suggested, many people who face infertility feel alienated in churches but still wish to belong to a supportive community. The RESOLVE chapter I studied more or less saw itself as purposefully filling that role. One newsletter article contrasted what RESOLVE can offer (unconditional support) with what religion can offer.[45] One copresident even referred to her leadership on different occasions as her "ministry" and "vocation." Even though they must follow the official positions of national RESOLVE and are subject to a great deal of influence from the infertility industry, local RESOLVE meetings provided a place for collective meaning making, especially during the more intimate peer discussions that comprised the first hour of every meeting. As one speaker from the Atlanta Center for Social Therapy pointed out, RESOLVE meetings are a "performance" in the sense of an entity formed by the people who attend, a group of people who come together and create what happens there.[46]

Whatever else they may or may not have done well, these discussions provided a space for challenging the myth of control and even for questioning consumerism, as if one could buy one's way out of the problem of infertility. People learned and were changed by confronting physical, technological, financial, and existential limits. They also learned from compassionate fellow sufferers, past and present, that life after infertility includes greater possibilities than people might initially have thought.

A Wider Generativity

Generally speaking, the experience of infertility, including treatments, presses people to figure out what they value: bodily health and well-being and important personal relationships, particularly with one's spouse but also with children they can nurture and love who may or may not be biologically related to their parents. Even while RESOLVE did not sufficiently challenge the idea that one ought to try at least some treatment, many contributors to these monthly discussions embraced what could be called a wider generativity. In other words, they believed life includes more than conceiving a child. Not only is there one's own life and health, but there is also the valued relationship with one's spouse/partner. There are also numerous ways to contribute to the lives of children and the wider world that can be generative.

In addition to the "Welcome to Holland" parable, people told each other another cautionary tale at RESOLVE meetings. The story may have started as a case from someone's psychotherapy practice, but it had become more of an urban legend by the time I heard it. According to the tale, a couple divorced after having a child through ART. The wife apparently had moved ahead with treatment without really getting her husband's full consent and cooperation. She, like many women facing infertility, did most of the research about treatment options and aggressively pursued cycle after cycle of IVF until a baby resulted. She was so single-minded in achieving her goal, in obtaining the coveted object, that she neglected her husband's wishes and neglected the marital relationship itself. The discussion leader who told the first version of the story I heard quoted the husband as saying, "Somewhere along the line, I lost her." According to the leader, the moral of the story was that "A lot of people have the child but are not at peace." She continued, "It is a sad commentary that we think this little child is going to provide that peace. You need to tend to the journey along the way."[47]

This message of embracing a wider generativity leads to two conclusions. The first pertains to the importance of developing personal virtues that replace the desire to control every aspect of life. The second pertains to the ultimately individualistic nature of this personal transformation. With regard to the first conclusion, the narratives of transformation and meaning making that emerged in RESOLVE, especially for people on the other side of infertility, contrasted sharply with the rhetoric of control heard frequently from people in the early stages of the infertility journey. Whatever cultural values people brought with them to RESOLVE meetings, the crisis of infertility seemed to initiate an epiphanic liberation in which people reevaluated themselves and their life plans, rediscovered interdependencies, and were forced to cultivate other virtues in addition to control. "Resolving" infertility required not necessarily having a child but "tending to the journey along the way."

With regard to the second conclusion, the values and virtues people rediscovered seemingly remained largely individualistic. The wider generativity preached by therapists and discussion leaders was still rather limited in scope, relating most directly to each person's life, spouse, and personal aspirations. There was no concern for the larger social context in which RESOLVE members found themselves. RESOLVE members were adept at the second phase of suffering, attending compassionately to each other's suffering through individual storytelling, but were less inclined to find a way to stand in solidarity against the conditions that exacerbate infertility, that make family life difficult for so many people, or that contribute to unjust social structures (all corresponding to the third phase of suffering). Most of all, they tended not to question enough why ART has to be the crucible out of which selves reemerge, with or without children.

Dorothee Soelle argues in *Suffering* (1975) that capitalism impedes viewing problems collectively and that a prerequisite for working on suffering is the conviction that we live in a world that can be changed.[48] Her insight resonates with my concerns about consumerist individualism, an orientation to the problem of infertility that impedes critical reflection on the infertility industry and the conditions that give rise to some kinds of infertility. People in RESOLVE, however compassionate they were with each other at meetings, were not inclined to view their problems collectively, in solidarity with others outside of RESOLVE, or to embrace the conviction that they lived in a world that could be changed. Indeed, when pressed to see their problems collectively, they resisted. On one occasion, two guest lecturers from the Atlanta Center for Social Therapy tried to get participants in the meeting to engage in group activities, building on the idea of RESOLVE as "performance" and the power of performative activities to bring about change. The group flatly rejected these activities, preferring instead to revert to the normal pattern of individual story sharing—or what seemed like individual therapy in a group setting.[49] They wanted to tell their stories, to talk and be listened to, and to "sit there and learn."[50] A potential opportunity for solidarity and social change was missed, I believe, when group members remained in an individualistic framework even when imagining a life after infertility that is wider than biological conception.

The Interests of Children, Parents, and Future Generations

Differences exist between ethicists' meaning making and actual infertility sufferers' meaning making about the value of children, the good of family, and our obligations to future generations. I intend this section to be dialogical as a way of suggesting what can be learned on both sides.

From the beginning of this project, I sought to explore the ways ART presses us to define how we value children, what we mean by the good(s) of family, and how we understand our relationship to future generations. This interest led me to pay particular attention to individuals' experiences with egg donation, preferences regarding disclosure to children of their biological origins, and descriptions of the experience of parenting after infertility.

Although my appraisal may contradict what many scholars have feared would be the logical consequence of ART, the people I observed did not, by and large, approach assisted reproduction as some frivolous personal project. They wanted to be parents and believed they would make good parents. They desired the parent-child relationship more than they coveted an object or a "designer baby." They felt punished and profoundly left out of one of life's most basic processes. These people also, by and large, gave a lot of thought to the issue of biological versus social parenting. Many of them struggled with interpreting the significance of severing the genetic tie to one parent, for example, and weighed carefully the difference between choosing adoption versus choosing an egg or sperm donor. Some fell back on the rhetoric of choice, believing this to be another area best left to private conscience and psychotherapy. But to be fair, much more reflection about the goods of family took place than some scholarly discussions of ART recognize.

If people say, based on their own experiences, that "it doesn't matter where the egg comes from," that the experience of pregnancy mitigates the absence of a genetic connection between mother and child, or that the experience of parenting somehow eclipses altogether the child's biological origins, ethicists ought to take these statements seriously and explore them more deeply. Maybe some of the presuppositions were faulty. Do "ideal" connections exist among genetic, gestational, and social parenthood? On what are they based? How much weight, if any, should be given to the biological? Conversely, if people who use ART have difficulty articulating what a future child's interests might be, then they need to be challenged to think more critically about the child's point of view. They may be taking risks on behalf of future children and future generations for which they can never be held fully accountable.

Making versus Begetting Children

Oliver O'Donovan predicted in *Begotten or Made?* (1984) that the use of reproductive technologies would fundamentally alter how people viewed children: they would be viewed as personal projects rather than beings of equal moral status with their parents.[51] He contrasted the activity of "making" (*poesis*) with the activity of "begetting" (*praxis*), a contrast that remains relevant in light of the acronym "ART" and prevalent construction metaphors, such as "family building." "Making" children, according to O'Donovan, would gradually and insidiously devalue the enterprise of procreation and would result in offspring who were not respected and loved as their naturally conceived parents had been. By forgetting that we are all begotten (that is, begotten by God), we would lose a sense of fundamental equality.

More recent ethical analyses of ART have expressed very similar concerns, although in place of an explicitly theological analysis are now critiques of ART based on the morally unsavory "commodification" of children that is perceived to result from the practice of buying and selling gametes and embryos, for example.[52] Children and the biological material needed to create them should not be subjected to market norms, many observers argue, because commodification diminishes their personhood and humanity. The essence of this humanity, if not explicitly contained within a theological framework, remains rooted in an ontology about what it means to be human. In secular philosophical arguments, to be fully human is to exist independently of another's designs or wishes.[53] Being human is to possess the capacity to develop autonomy and to possess outright inalienable rights that all humans share. This quality of what it means to be human at times is articulated in terms of a child's right to an "open future."[54]

Whether one looks to religious or philosophical ethics, an ongoing scholarly debate questions how we value children in general and children born via reproductive or genetic technologies in particular. My research may not allay ethicists' concerns about commodification but should complicate them somewhat. The tendency to speak of the expense of ART as equivalent to a new house or car or vacation and the practice of selecting egg and sperm donors by picking traits for one's offspring from a catalog of choices (as in the case of the clinic rep who claimed her patient told her, "I gotta have a Michelle Pfeiffer")[55] are two examples that suggest a consumeristic approach to childbearing but not necessarily a guarantee that the children born from these procedures will be viewed as consumer items. In fact, in terms of what was publicly shared during meetings, I heard only the most traditional expressions of unconditional love for children conceived by ART or adopted. What may start out looking like commodification may not end up as the actual commodification of children—not when the fantasy of a child becomes a human being whose existence depends on devoted and continuous care.

In addition, my research with this group of people in Atlanta suggests that the stories of American couples paying fifty thousand dollars for an egg donor represent the exception rather than the rule. Such extreme examples of commodification depict a wildly distant scenario from the everyday use of fertility treatments that were discussed at RESOLVE meetings. The people I met were not looking for designer babies; they just wanted to be parents. In fact, they did not turn quickly and easily to third-party donation despite the strong and favorable messages they received from clinics and physicians who specialized in egg donation.

In general, the people I observed gave a great deal of thought to having and parenting children. By necessity, they had to be more intentional and deliberate about their values than was the case for fertile people. For example, the home study a couple must complete before adopting a child is an exceptionally thorough investigation of the couple's readiness for parenthood and their values about child rearing. Couples also took the choice between adoption and third-party donation very seriously, recognizing it as an occasion to specify what is owed to children. "Why are we producing this child when others need homes?,"[56] one woman asked rhetorically, recounting her decision to adopt.

I think RESOLVE members asked themselves, in their own words, whether creating children through ART promotes human flourishing. For example, what does the discussion about whether to disclose to children the nature of their origins say about what they thought to be the most important ethical issue? I think their overriding concern with the merits of disclosure versus secrecy suggests that these aspiring parents cared deeply about the interests of their future children. They were not focused exclusively on childbearing as a self-referential project; their attention was already focused on the child in anticipation of what that potential future child would need. Of primary concern was that their potential future children be treated like other children and have a solid sense of identity. Although alternative interpretations are certainly possible, I think these concerns challenge the presumption that children born through ART are inherently "objectified" or "commodified." Even if the initial impulse was to approach ART like a consumer item, this was not a persisting or overriding attitude in the individuals I observed. RESOLVE members, like most people, hoped to be good parents.

Ethicists often raise the concern that the quest for a genetic tie to a child through ART can seem to deemphasize the importance of social parenting. Dorothy Roberts argues that the use of ART is motivated by the desire for racial purity, to make sure the genes of white parents are passed on.[57] Lisa Cahill and Elizabeth Bartholet claim that the relative availability and allure of ART undermines the likelihood of adoption.[58] However, the use of ART can also signify the opposite emphasis: social parenting taking precedence over biological ties. When a couple uses a donor, after all, one parent is saying he or she can live without a biological connection to the child.

The people I observed seemed to have less, not more, conventional views of what counts as a family. What matters is having a family, not having the perfect dream child, and prior to that, what matters is taking care of the marriage relationship or partnership.[59] Participants at the meetings I observed, however, maintained a conspicuous silence on the issue of homosexual partnerships. No statements were made against them at any level, but no homosexual couples attended the meetings. The values that were expressed would seem to imply acceptance of homosexual parents, but the group was never tested on this point. Group members did clearly articulate the idea that members of a family ought to be committed to each other's well-being: a family need not be a group of people who are related genetically, and a family need not be any bigger than two people, but however many members a family has, they need to care about each other. Such a definition of "family" closely resembles Iris Marion Young's description: "I define family as people who live together and/or share resources necessary to the means of life and comfort; who are committed to taking care of one another's physical and emotional needs to the best of their ability; who conceive themselves in a relatively long-term, if not permanent, relationship; and who recognize themselves as family. . . . Family entails commitment and obligation as well as comfort: family members make claims on one another that they do not make on others."[60] The openness in group discussions toward third-party donation cohered with the group's open-minded view of the family more generally.

The question of whether ART deemphasizes or reemphasizes the importance of social parenting can be illuminated by looking at what ethical theory leads us to expect about the impact of severing biological and social parenting and what experience tells us about this disconnection in actuality. For example, what does it mean that people say, "It doesn't matter where the egg comes from?" What weight or privilege should this statement receive? Although I may not be able to answer these questions definitively, I firmly believe that ethicists need at least to hear such statements and reflect critically on normative assumptions.

As discussed earlier, Cahill objects to third-party donors of eggs or sperm in ART procedures in part because she believes that the introduction of a third party into the marriage relationship will disrupt the unity of biological, gestational, and social parenting. In Cahill's view, this disruption does not benefit women and men but presents serious ethical problems. First and foremost, it privileges the "voluntary and intersubjective meanings of sex, marriage, and parenthood" above the biological ones. Cahill explains her point of view using the example of artificial insemination, saying that the "basic difference between" using the husband's sperm and that of a donor "is that the latter sever[s] key physical relationships . . . , thus denying them any significant moral weight."[61]

In severing these physical relationships, use of either an egg donor or a sperm donor also creates an asymmetrical relationship between the husband and wife and their child that could damage both the marriage and the parents' relationship with their child. Cahill insists that a couple's "unity as spouses" is more important than one spouse realizing her/his physical reproductive potential without the other: "There is a natural unity of the intentional and physical dimensions of spousehood and parenthood which should not be broken deliberately."[62]

Disrupting the unity among biological, gestational, and social parenting also puts children's welfare at risk, according to Cahill. She is skeptical about the unknown, long-range impact of assisted reproduction on children's identity and selfhood. Drawing on what adopted children have reported about their experience, Cahill claims that "corporeal bonds are important to our identities as human beings."[63] She cautions against prioritizing adult "need fulfillment" over child welfare when creating a child through assisted reproduction rather than adopting one already in existence.

The lived reality raises questions about the validity of Cahill's claims, however. As far as I could discern, RESOLVE members deeply valued the marriage relationship. This value was articulated most explicitly during the Valentine's Day meeting, which focused all of its advice on maintaining couples' well-being during infertility. Couples were also frequently admonished to be "on the same page" in their decision making, to respect each other's feelings, and to make important choices together. However, mutual respect between spouses was not assumed to require literal symmetry in the relationship of each parent to the child. People very much honored mutuality and equality but did not embrace "symmetry" as Cahill defines it. What does that say about what they valued or what weight the body or biological received?

In addressing the RESOLVE group during a formal presentation, the woman who had become pregnant with her younger sister's eggs claimed that her daughter's biological origins made absolutely no difference in how she and her husband related to their child. They emphasized that although they intended to explain to their daughter how she was conceived and had already begun explaining the story in age-appropriate terms, in their eyes the significance of the egg donation was only diminishing with time. The more time they had with their daughter, the less and less it seemed to matter how she had been conceived.

What about the experience of being pregnant made one woman claim that it "doesn't matter where the egg comes from?" What about the experience of becoming parents made this couple's experience with egg donation so positive? Should these claims be trusted? I think it would be naive to accept these claims uncritically, especially given the powerful forces that keep people on the treadmill of infertility until something works. Nevertheless, such claims deserve to be taken seriously. Generally speaking, children born through these procedures are deeply wanted and loved—perhaps more than many other children. One of RESOLVE's mottos—"All babies are precious, RESOLVE babies are the most precious"—speaks to this intense devotion. These parents also are privy to bodily and experiential knowledge that runs counter to what theorists predicted in the abstract. Ultimately, though, the most enlightening answers will have to come from the children of ART, when they are old enough to respond directly to the question of whether the source of the egg (or sperm) matters to them. Only then will we have a good idea whether any real harm has been done.

Future Generations and the Common Good

Very few long-range studies can tell us anything about the psychological well-being of children conceived through the use of third-party donors. In addition, there are no guarantees that information about donors will be available in the future when these children need or want to obtain it. Although discussion participants expressed a lot of anxiety about the long-term consequences of egg/sperm donation, discussion leaders and clinic representatives usually allayed these concerns by claiming that such practices would only become more common. Their attitude toward children's future need for information about donors seemed somewhat cavalier, and their confidence in the lasting power of the clinics that employed them was unwarranted. They also neglected to address the possibility that half-siblings might meet and attempt to have children without knowing of their biological relationship and of potential regulation of clinics to prevent such occurrences. We are not, I believe, thinking enough about future consequences and future children.

Conversely, I appreciate that ART challenges traditional views of identity that depend on one mother, one father, and a knowable family history through each. It is impossible to predict the identity of a child who has had as many as five or more adults contribute to his or her genetic/gestational/social parenting.[64] Some strands of feminist theory would view these challenges to customary ways of thinking about selfhood as positive developments because they foster the idea that all selves are constituted from multiple sources.[65] If the use of third-party donors fostered greater respect for nontraditional families and reemphasized the importance of social parenting and the underlying commitment to each partner's well-being as the definition of family, then I would also embrace this use of ART as a positive development.

For the family of a child born through egg or sperm donation, the focus ideally becomes the present and future well-being of that particular child and the parents' love for him or her. The social relationship of the present receives more weight than the genetic heritage of the past. Thus, a child born through egg or sperm donation could ideally be expected to adjust to the knowledge of his or her origins in much the same way as a child adopted into a healthy and loving family. Some RESOLVE discussion leaders argued that adjusting to the knowledge of being born from a donor gamete is easier than adjusting to the knowledge of being adopted: in the first case, a woman made a generous donation of eggs—more akin to a blood donation, it was reasoned—to another woman who needed them. In the second case, a mother (and father) relinquished the child at birth. One discussion leader gave the example of a couple who had put their third baby (resulting from an unplanned pregnancy) up for adoption because they had wanted only two children. How much more difficult for that child, people surmised with some horror, than for the child born from a generous third-party donation.

Although it remains plausible that children born from egg/sperm donation will fare better than children who are adopted, this idea constitutes no more than untested speculation. The proponents of egg donation, particularly the clinic representatives who came to RESOLVE to tout the benefits of egg donation for older women, seemed to be making many assumptions about what future children's experiences will be like, assumptions that should be more carefully scrutinized and that would benefit from more sustained ethical reflection. By this I mean something more substantial than "What would you have wanted your parents to tell you about your biological heritage?" The issue of disclosure, though important, does not cover all that is potentially problematic about third-party donation. Because an irreducible presumption always arises in claiming on children's behalf what will best serve their future interests (and the claim is suspiciously self-serving for adults looking to rationalize the use of third-party donors), I think we need to ask harder questions and collect more data.

Finally, in addition to concerns about the health and well-being of children and generations not yet born, the well-being of adult women who currently use ART must be considered. It remains an open question why ART needs to be a part of their transformation process in resolving infertility. One RESOLVE leader, who decided with her husband to be child-free after many years of infertility treatment, opened the door to considering this question. "My husband wanted me to stay on fertility drugs for the rest of my life, because that was hope," she said. "Despite the trauma and expense of the high-tech stuff, there's always the hope of having a biological child. When you first start, . . . everybody longs for that biological child. As long as there's one more treatment, there's hope that it will work. When it doesn't work, what happens to your hope?"[66] In the course of the discussion, she suggested that ART "postpones the final chapter" of the infertility process and thus postpones the disappointment. But she did not address and no one in the group considered the great costs of this postponement: the personal expense to individuals, both financial and emotional; the health risks, particularly for women, of treatment; and the general impact on the common good.

Looking Ahead

Ethics needs to attend to the voices of the infertile. It needs to pay attention to the bodily knowledge obtained from the experience of infertility and undergoing infertility treatments. Ethics cannot answer some questions without attending to personal experience, including whether a child's method of conception makes an emotional and psychological difference in that child's life and that of his or her parents—or, more generally, what differences arise as a consequence of a child's method of arrival in the family that is now raising him or her. Likewise, people in RESOLVE are not asking some questions of themselves that I believe they should. Foremost among these questions is the impact of ART on the health and well-being of women and children and future generations. The analogy between egg donation and blood donation seems weak and unsubstantiated because we cannot assume that children born from these procedures will not assign at least some weight to the genetic heritage from which they were disconnected.

Were ethical treatments of ART to become more nuanced in their assessment of this technology and more sophisticated in their understanding of

ART's role in the larger journey of infertility, people facing infertility—or at least the people I observed in RESOLVE—likely might become more open to engaging in explicitly ethical analysis about the use of ART.

Ultimately, though, an organization such as RESOLVE bears a special responsibility to foster more critical reflection, especially about the larger social context, so that people can step off the treadmill when they need or want to do so. Some force in society must connect these individual experiences back to the level of a concern for the common good, and RESOLVE could play this role.

Conclusion

Implications for Policy

My interpretation of assisted reproductive technologies (ART), based on a year of listening carefully to the voices of women and their partners who were using such technologies, is that they often served an important purpose beyond the obvious goal of trying to become pregnant. Regardless of whether ART led to the birth of a healthy child, the process of undergoing rounds of in vitro fertilization (IVF) often served in part as a ritual—a consumeristic ritual —that aided people in working through the grief of infertility. People seemed to feel a need to try ART, even when they knew their chances of success were very low, so that they could feel as if they were "doing something" to solve their problem. If anything, the physical difficulty and expense of IVF trials enhanced the value of going through them; they were a brutal workout—both physical and spiritual—with a high potential payoff.

The large and lucrative infertility industry that strives to make this technology readily available—at least to those who can afford it—taps into people's desire to be "doing something." By my observation, only very rarely did people who had the financial means to try ART voluntarily choose to forgo it and instead move directly to adopting a child or deciding to live child-free. More often, people seemed to follow a predictable progression: first low-tech infertility treatment, then ART, then ART with a donor gamete (if applicable), then resolution through adoption or through deciding to be child-free.

Throughout this process, very little stood in the way of destructive over-consumption of ART. In 2007, the infertility industry remains largely unregulated—or, more precisely, it is regulated by a patchwork of direct and indirect government measures combined with the self-policing of individual doctors and clinics. In the United States, there are no recommended or uniformly imposed limits on how many rounds of IVF a woman can try, how many embryos may be implanted in a woman's uterus at once, or how much a donor may charge for her eggs. What limits exist are set largely by the for-profit clinics themselves and more often pertain to who may try what procedure, such as age limits for women trying IVF with their own eggs. Physicians may or may not counsel restraint, so individuals are largely left on their own to decide when enough is enough. Sometimes limit setting derives only from a lack of insurance, insufficient personal financial resources, or the support and counsel of a therapist or fellow member of a group such as RESOLVE.

ART procedures have never had to pass through the kinds of clinical trials that are required of new drugs and devices. Eggs and sperm are not "devices," and the drugs used in IVF were originally approved for other purposes. No long-term studies have tracked the safety of multiple exposures to the powerful drugs used during IVF, and very few studies have tracked the health of children born through ART. In other words, the women undergoing these procedures and the children born from them constitute the primary experimental trial.

Despite the lack of careful study, ART has been routinized to the point where it is offered and accepted as a legitimate medical option without much question. As with the many increasingly sophisticated methods that enable pregnant women to detect fetal abnormalities, assisted reproductive technologies now have the force of a technological mandate. They are the latest and most effective means for solving the medical problem of infertility. Physicians offer IVF just as they offer repeated ultrasounds to pregnant women, epidurals to women in labor, and elective Caesarean sections—because these technologies are available and patients demand them. However, as Rayna Rapp has pointed out in her ethnographic account of amniocentesis in the United States, these technologies often require individuals to be "moral pioneers."[1] In the rush to provide services to patients, individuals remain on their own to weigh competing values and make judgments. In the case of prenatal testing, for example, a woman might be offered the latest screening technique as a matter of routine (especially if she is over thirty-five) but given no guidance or education about what living with a particular disability in her child would be like. Only the unspoken but obvious implication of terminating the pregnancy will be on the table.[2] With assisted reproduction, the high-tech options might be offered as soon as they are indicated medically, but the individual is on her own to navigate privately through the moral implications of various reproductive decisions. Absent is a thorough examination of the ends of ART and the ends of medicine: for example, whether doctors ought to be offering repeated IVF trials as part of good medical practice or whether the conception of a child with donor gametes is a good and worthy goal.

The justification for ART, as with all quasi-elective medical procedures, lies most fundamentally in the value of autonomous patient choice. I do not disagree that individuals are best suited to decide for themselves what risks to accept and what values are important in the area of reproduction. But the rhetoric of choice belies the coercive pressures that can develop in a free market for ART. The infertility industry generates $4 billion a year, and the market for ART has the potential to expand dramatically as more insurance plans begin to mandate at least partial coverage of infertility treatments.[3] I believe it is disingenuous to defer to individual patient "choice" when so much money may be made on the backs (or wombs) of women who use ART. After completing my research, I question even more strenuously whether America's essentially laissez-faire approach to reproductive technologies truly serves patients' best interests. Individual women get stuck on the treadmill of infertility the same way most Americans get stuck in Juliet Schor's so-called squirrel cage of capitalism: the more they get of what they think they want, the more they need.

The United States is anomalous among countries that have access to reproductive technologies in not imposing uniform federal restrictions. Policymakers must recognize that the infertility industry needs greater regulation and oversight both as a matter of ethics and as a matter of public health. The President's Council on Bioethics called for greater regulation of the infertility industry in its 2004 report, *Reproduction and Responsibility*. Unfortunately, the substance of that valuable report has been obscured by various political agendas, including the facile polarization of the public debate around the issue of freedom of choice. Any suggestion that individuals' choices be curtailed in the area of reproduction is usually portrayed as antithetical to freedom and the American way of life.

Organizations such as RESOLVE could play a very important role in lobbying for key policy changes, including scientific studies of the long-term impact of IVF drugs, scientific studies of the health of babies born through ART, psychological studies of children born through the use of third-party gamete donors, regulation of clinic practices and the financing of ART, regulation of donor selection and pricing, and many more areas. RESOLVE occupies a unique position: it has earned both the trust of its members and the respect of the infertility industry. As I have suggested, this dual loyalty can and does create potential conflicts of interest. RESOLVE could also choose to critique how well it is meeting its stated mission of support for the infertile and could examine more closely what this support should look like. It could take advantage of its unique position as both a neutral nonprofit "above the fray" and a highly professionalized mainstream organization very much entwined with the infertility industry. It could use its credibility to exert some influence in both domains—with patients and with industry—and make significant changes in the way people use ART in the United States.

To remain a credible advocate for the infertile, RESOLVE should have higher ambitions than simply protecting options for the sake of options. RESOLVE should more explicitly and publicly examine the purpose of ART: Is it really a treatment for the illness of infertility, as the group's leaders claim, or is ART better thought of as an elective procedure that legitimately expresses procreative liberty. These purposes are not mutually exclusive, but insofar as RESOLVE unwittingly reinforces the logic of unlimited procreative liberty or the "ideology of choice" in its policy statements and in its actions, it does nothing to restrain the overconsumption of ART. To remain a credible advocate for the infertile, RESOLVE should also examine its high prioritization of mandated health insurance coverage for infertility services. To what degree does the group's relationship with the infertility industry drive that prioritization? If mandating health insurance coverage for ART has the unintended consequence of enabling couples to undertake futile or nearly futile treatments, then it arguably does more harm than good.

These recommendations for RESOLVE are intended as constructive and do not detract from RESOLVE's many benefits, including the tremendous support it offers to its members: on the local level, it even ostensibly serves as a substitute church for suffering people who seek out genuine community with compassionate others. RESOLVE does a great service to its members by providing a forum in which they can connect and a space where people can feel safe from judgment. Nevertheless, RESOLVE should strive to be more than a group of "balcony people" for individuals struggling with decisions about ART. It can and should play a more prophetic role, challenging its members and society at large to question whether ART has become a consumeristic ritual and suggesting ways to step off the treadmill. RESOLVE's diverse and wise membership can help put the experience of infertility and our responses to it into the context of a wider perspective.

So, although I suggest that RESOLVE is implicated to some degree in the overconsumption of ART, I also believe that it provides the space and possesses the resources to challenge the larger social and economic causes of this problem.

Implications for Ethics

If anything is clear after the completion of my research and in light of developments since I began this project, it is that ethics needs the social sciences.

Ethical analysis of ART and the conditions that give rise to its use cannot legitimately progress without studying the real-life experience of infertility. I chose to immerse myself for a year in the social world of RESOLVE. I could have made other choices. I could have shadowed individuals through the course of their treatment at a fertility clinic. I could have studied an explicitly religious support group, such as Hannah's Prayer. I could have researched the growing world of Internet support networks. Each of these choices would naturally have highlighted certain angles, such as the doctor-patient relationship, the role of faith, or the cyberworld of social interaction. My decision had its limitations, but it gave me one snapshot, one window, into the use of ART in the southern United States at the very beginning of the twenty-first century. Because of RESOLVE's presence in the nation's capital as a lobbying organization and because of its function on the local level as a public forum, the choice highlighted the political context and contested notions of justice, individual freedom, procreative liberty, and duties to the common good.

I conducted my final in-person interview for this project on the morning of September 11, 2001, in an Atlanta coffee shop. I met with a woman who had been attending RESOLVE meetings to learn about options for dealing with her infertility. I was newly pregnant with my second child, fighting nausea, and concerned that my interviewee not learn of my pregnancy. We cut short the interview when my husband called to tell me that the first World Trade Center tower had fallen. In a follow-up phone interview several days later, this woman admitted that she felt confused and ambivalent about her plans to have a child: whether she could procreate seemed insignificant in the face of national and international events.

Since 2001, most Americans have moved on with their everyday lives, including the business of having babies. The infertility industry has grown steadily, as has the public debate about ART. The media frequently covers the issue of "designer babies" and often features debates between scholars on the ethics of pre-conception sex selection, preimplantation genetic diagnosis, and other technologies that may someday allow prospective parents to control various aspects of their children's genetic makeup. This continued public interest in ART and related technologies has coexisted with the ever-present "abortion wars" in all their guises.[4] The deeply conservative Bush administration, which prides itself on embodying the so-called culture of life, has gone out of its way to fuel the acrimony that exists around the abortion issue. In all of these topics, which raise a host of ethical issues, it has been too easy to oversimplify, to rely on untested assumptions, and to instrumentalize individuals' experiences for political purposes.

It thus becomes evident that ethics needs the social sciences first and foremost as a check. Hindsight can also provide a correction for misguided theories and judgments, but hindsight often comes too late. Christine Rosen's recent historical work has described in vivid detail the enthusiasm with which American clergy embraced the eugenics movement of the early twentieth century, for example.[5] Protestant ministers around the country competed with each other to write compelling sermons preaching the virtues of eugenics, becoming adept at using Christian Scripture to support their arguments, including the idea that weeding out society's weaker elements constituted an act of Christian charity. Their sermons drew support from the most progressive, proscience elements of American society at the time and resonated with judgments coming down from the highest court in the land: "Three generations of imbeciles," after all, were "enough."[6] Unfortunately, one consequence of the American eugenics movement was the forcible sterilization of tens of thousands of individuals deemed "feebleminded" or otherwise unfit to reproduce. Over four decades, these legal, state-sanctioned sterilizations increasingly targeted black women; the sterilizations were not halted until the 1970s.

The example of the American eugenics movement demonstrates, among other things, that scholars, judges, and clergy can be wrong. People who claim the authority of their religion can be wrong. People can be persuaded by ideas in the abstract that have little basis in fact, and the public can go along with unchallenged ideas for a very long time before any change occurs. To be responsible, ethics, including Christian ethics, must be open to new information and open to correction. If our argument for increased access to ART is based on justice, we must ask, justice for whom and according to what values? Mandated health insurance coverage for ART only helps those people with health insurance; it does nothing for those Americans who both lack insurance and suffer from infertility. If our argument against the use of donor eggs and sperm to conceive children is based on notions of human flourishing, backed by the authority of religion, we must ask, flourishing for whom and according to what values? It is not self-evident that certain choices or certain uses of technologies will be contrary to human flourishing or disrespectful to some amorphous notion of a "culture of life." These arguments must receive substantial elaboration and clarification and should be forced to reckon with complex realities that may push back against them.

The methodological dimensions of this project—that is, the incorporation of social science methods into ethical analysis—sought to reckon with the complex reality of infertility. The many months of research that produced the ethnographic account for this book did not take place in a library but in a hospital auditorium, in coffee shops, and over the phone in conversations with real people who had endured or were enduring incredibly physically, economically, and spiritually demanding times. Reckoning with the lived experience of infertility required revising some of my starting assumptions. It required a greater sense of compassion for the people I was studying as well as closer scrutiny of my values. Without losing sight of the original concerns that motivated me, I had to admit that many of the people I encountered believed that ethical critiques of ART were not only irrelevant to the decisions they were making but also downright offensive. I had to contemplate the possibility that perhaps the ethical critiques that seemed so persuasive to me in the abstract were indeed irrelevant or at least in need of considerable revision. I ultimately remained unconvinced that ethical critique should be avoided out of deference to the alleged moral neutrality of RESOLVE. But to be effective and useful,[7] any ethical analysis I made needed to tread carefully and respectfully.

Most people struggling with infertility, I found, are not trying to have "designer babies." They are not paying tens of thousands of dollars for a premium donor egg. They are not interested in interfering with anyone else's plans to have a child, nor do they want anyone else to interfere with their plans. They want for themselves what they perceive other regular people want: a healthy child to raise and love. It is a mundane but profound and some would say universal desire.

Despite my sympathy for individuals struggling with infertility, I believe it would be a serious mistake to abandon the use of ART to the ideology of choice and thereby avoid asking difficult normative questions. Too much is at stake in this social practice, including the health and well-being of women and families and future generations of children. We need more explicit examination of the values that drive social practices and policies. Why, for example, are some children called into existence through years of effort and expense at the same time that others spend their childhoods adrift from families, waiting for adoption? Are justice and human freedom truly honored? Why are some women and not others encouraged to reproduce? Are we intensifying class and race privileges or even inaugurating a new age of American eugenics? An individual facing the decision to try IVF may be in no condition to contemplate these questions, but they are not beyond what RESOLVE as an organization could consider or what the public debate should more generally encompass.

Final Thoughts on RESOLVE

RESOLVE misses a tremendous opportunity by forsaking more explicitly normative conversation. Ethics, including religious ethics, has not been welcome in this setting because it has been perceived as one more source of stigmatizing judgment. However, people in an organization such as RESOLVE would benefit from what normative discussion can offer: the vocabulary for moving the conversation outside an individualistic framework, which frequently serves only the interests of the infertility industry, to a larger perspective that helps people consider and reflect on their connections with other individuals, with social structures, and with the common good. Without the language and ideas of ethics, people may have difficulty resisting the pressures to use ART that begin for many with the work-family conflict and delayed childbearing and are then fed by consumerism. Without the language and ideas of ethics, people may find it impossible to see beyond their own narrow interests as defined by their socioeconomic class, race, gender, and even geography. Having a baby becomes the whole world, which, although entirely understandable, seems like a distortion of human flourishing and a subversion of the common good.

Although the narratives of transformation told and retold in RESOLVE meetings constitute important and creative acts of meaning making and provide constructive tools for enduring grief, they often do little to encourage individuals to stand in solidarity against the conditions that at least in part have led them to this place: the ineluctable "need" to try everything possible before infertility can be successfully resolved. Talking openly and normatively about the many ethical dimensions of ART could empower people to exercise more reflective self-determination in responding to the personal crisis of infertility as well as the social context in which it occurs.

As Judith Shklar reminds us, how a society responds to the "natural" occurrences of human existence, such as the more limited window of female fertility, says a great deal about its ideals of justice.[8] We have the power to make the experience of pregnancy, of balancing work and family, and of infertility sources of women's oppression by the social structures we institute or fail to institute; we also have the power to work to create the conditions for justice. We possess the power to shape aspects of our social world. But we are not all-powerful. We live within the confines of certain times and places, with external constraints bearing down on all our choices. Yet even granting these constraints, we can still say that better and worse choices exist in the area of reproduction. Some choices promise to promote human flourishing where others threaten to undermine it.

This book does not offer a simple answer to the question of what moral weight ought to be given to biological ties to one's child and whether the use of third-party donors inevitably disrupts parent-child bonds and generally undermines human flourishing. The experience of adoption, as described by numerous members of RESOLVE, strongly suggests that the biological tie is not at all determinative of family goods. Yet the case of egg/sperm donors is more ambiguous and raises precisely the kinds of questions that need greater input from both ethics and experience. We will never come to an adequate assessment of third-party donors until we expand and deepen the conversation about ART and its impact on the well-being of children and families. I believe that ethical analyses can maintain a social perspective while still honoring the richness of individual experience, the reality of suffering, the difficulty of decision making, and legitimacy of individual agency. On this subject, as on others, ethics and experience can and must speak to each other.

Methodological
Afterword

Specific Methodological Choices

A Case Study

This book is a case study of the use of assisted reproductive technologies (ART) in the United States, based on the experiences of people who attended the monthly meetings of a local chapter of RESOLVE (RESOLVE of Georgia) during the 2000–2001 program year. By case study, I mean an in-depth qualitative analysis of a single group of people that involved personal interaction, observation, and interviews. I did not survey the members of this RESOLVE chapter, nor did I compare this particular group of RESOLVE members against other chapters across the country, of which there are more than fifty. I also did not compare in any systematic way the experiences of people within the group I observed against people in other kinds of support groups (for example, Hannah's Prayer) or against the general population of individuals who experience infertility.

I sought to immerse myself in a particular group of individuals in a particular time and place and learn about their experiences with infertility and ART. My goal was to test the theoretical arguments outlined in chapter 1: primarily that ART functions as a technological fix for the social problem of delayed childbearing and that the use of ART is supported by an uncritical acceptance of procreative liberty. I chose this group as a critical case because RESOLVE supports the use of ART, is known for its support of ART, and is a powerful advocate for the infertile. By "critical case," I mean a case with strategic importance in relation to the general use of ART in this country. According to Bent Flyvbjerg, a critical case seeks "to achieve information which permits logical deductions of the type, 'if this is (not) valid for this case, then it applies to all (no) cases.'"[1] By choosing to study an environment that supports the use of ART, I hoped to discover whether these theoretical arguments were relevant and if so, in what ways. In other words, if these arguments were going to be relevant anywhere, they would likely be relevant in RESOLVE, whose members commonly use and accept ART. Moreover, if these arguments did not obtain in RESOLVE, they probably would not apply more generally. (For example, the argument that people who use ART do so because they have elected to delay childbearing is incomplete even in RESOLVE, where almost everyone tries ART. The reasons for using ART are more complex and center on the transformative process that derives from the consumeristic ritual of undergoing treatment.)

My research methods included participant observation, which involved writing detailed field notes; individual interviewing; and analyzing written materials provided by RESOLVE. I will now explain each of these aspects of my research.

Participant Observation

With the prior permission of RESOLVE leaders and after receiving approval for my research protocol from Emory University's Institutional Review Board, I attended the monthly meetings of a RESOLVE chapter for the program year running from September 2000 to May 2001. I observed a total of nine monthly meetings (which run about two to four hours) plus two all-day Saturday symposia, for an estimated minimum of forty hours of participant observation. Monthly meetings took place in classroom/auditorium space in an Atlanta-area hospital. Although monthly meetings are open to the public, nonmembers were charged a ten-dollar fee for attending. I formally joined RESOLVE during the year I was conducting my research, and group leaders were aware of my membership status at the time of my research.

RESOLVE's support group coordinator denied my request to attend private, therapist-led support groups held in members' homes. These support groups are for women and couples dealing with emotional issues surrounding infertility of all kinds. Members pay an average of thirty dollars per session and decide as a group how frequently to meet (typically every two or three weeks). In addition to these general infertility support groups, RESOLVE runs specialized therapist-led support groups in which the members meet to discuss specific issues (for example, miscarriage, secondary infertility, adoption, pregnancy after infertility, child-free living). Finally, more informal peer-led discussion groups are also open to members, free of charge, and take place in the home of a member ("hostess"). These are the "living room" discussion groups.

I requested permission only to attend the first of these types of support groups. After I had attended several monthly RESOLVE meetings and established a good rapport with leaders and attendees, my request to observe one of the private support groups might have been granted. However, I decided not to pursue the private support groups because the monthly meetings were so informative. They provided the opportunity to observe both peer discussion and formal presentations and tended to draw larger groups than the private support groups would have. More variety of attendees occurred from

Table A.1: Monthly Meetings and Saturday Symposia Attended, Noting Sponsors

Meetings	Date
"Celebrating Twenty Years of RESOLVE of Georgia: The Many Faces of RESOLVE . . . The Many Reasons for Hope"	September 2000
"Ask the Experts," sponsored by Reproductive Biology Associates of Atlanta and Organon, Inc.	October 2000
"Coping with the Holidays," sponsored by Concord Pharmacy	November 2000
"Counselors' Corner," sponsored by Atlanta Center for Reproductive Medicine	December 2000
"Navigating the Infertility Information Highway"	January 2001
Saturday Symposium: "Pathways to Adoptions"	February 2001
"Still Valentine's—Even after Infertility," sponsored by Organon, Inc.	February 2001
"Shattered Dreams: Dealing with Grief, Loss, and Anger," sponsored by Reproductive Biology Associates of Atlanta	March 2001
"The Medical, Financial, Legal, and Emotional Aspects of Using Donor Egg or Sperm or Surrogate," sponsored by Atlanta Center for Reproductive Medicine	April 2001
Saturday Symposium: "Mind/Body Retreat"	April 2001
"Disclosure: How Do We Tell Our Child/Children?"	May 2001

month to month, yet enough of a consistent core existed that I could see a group ethos at work. The monthly meetings also provided a window into RESOLVE's organizational dynamics as it is situated in the wider infertility industry as well as insight into the personal struggles of individuals and couples who attended.

In general, I was a silent observer, although discussion leaders always introduced me to the group and asked me to say a little bit about my research interests and my commitment to protecting confidentiality. Group members were always asked about their comfort level with my presence. In the early months of my research, this question was posed when I was not present. No one ever objected. As the year progressed and people in the group became familiar with my observation, leaders continued to ask group members about their comfort level with my presence but often did so in my presence. Some group members may not have felt free to object to my observation. But there are no circumstances in which I could have procured a "pure" and objective description of the group discussions. My presence as a researcher—silent or not—was a part of the dynamic of the discussion from the very beginning. (This dynamic manifested itself explicitly on a few occasions, as when the discussion leader asked me directly in the middle of a discussion whether I thought a relationship existed between infertility and "not having experienced a lot of failures" in other areas of life.)

Participant observation is a type of microanalysis of a social situation intended to have larger implications. The extended case method utilizes participant observation to test theoretical assumptions against a social world and then builds revised and more informed theory. Michael Burawoy's description of the extended case method suggests some of the benefits of this kind of analysis: "The importance of the single case lies in what it tells us about society as a whole rather than about the population of similar cases. . . . In constituting a social situation as unique, the extended case method pays attention to its complexity, its depth, its thickness. Causality then becomes multiplex, involving an 'individual' (i.e., undividable) connectedness of elements, tying the social situation to its context of determination."[2]

Field Notes

In conjunction with my participant observation, I wrote detailed field notes of every meeting I attended. I kept handwritten notes during the meetings and transcribed and elaborated these notes into written text as soon as possible thereafter.

I harbored no illusions about the purity of my descriptions but recognized that an interpretive dialectic is built into the process of writing notes. The qualitative data I derived were a product of my prior interpretive decisions. As Robert Emerson, Rachel Fretz, and Linda Shaw explain, "The ethnographer's assumptions, interests, and theoretical commitments enter into every phase of writing an ethnography and influence decisions that range from selecting which events to write about to those that entail emphasizing one member's perspective on an event over those of others. The process thus involves reflexive or dialectical interplay between theory and data whereby theory enters in at every point, shaping not only analysis but how social events come to be perceived and written up as data in the first place."[3] Although my field notes and the themes I compiled from them are driven by my prior agendas, I endeavored to provide enough detail to allow readers to come away with diverse interpretations.

Interviews

I supplemented my participant observation with nine semistructured interviews based on a set of standard questions but in which the discussion was flexible and responsive to the issues that arose. The interview schedule I used received approval from Emory's Institutional Review Board and appears in appendix B. Most of the interviews lasted well over an hour and were tape-recorded and transcribed. Five were phone interviews, three were face-to-face interviews, and one was conducted as a series of e-mail exchanges.

All of those I interviewed either currently were experiencing infertility or had experienced infertility in the past. Four interviews were conducted with RESOLVE organization leaders and/or speakers at the group's meetings. Eight of the inter-

Table A.2: Persons Interviewed, Noting Affiliation with RESOLVE

Persons Interviewed	Female	Male
Current or past leaders within local RESOLVE chapter	2	
Monthly meeting presenters / discussion leaders (trained therapists)	1	1
Current RESOLVE members and participants in monthly meeting discussions	3	
Non-RESOLVE members	2	

viewees were women. I focused primarily on women because ART is a constellation of procedures performed on women's bodies in an effort to become pregnant and women, therefore, are the most directly affected by the use of ART. However, because men were always present at RESOLVE meetings and because gender differences were a frequent topic of conversation, my focus widened to include how both women and men navigate infertility, not just the impact of this particular technology on women.

These interviews represent an opportunity sample. I did not set out with a particular plan for which people I would interview (for example, participant versus leader, member versus nonmember) but rather interviewed individuals as the occasion arose and / or they expressed interest in being interviewed.

Written Materials

I used many written materials in my research of RESOLVE at both the national and local levels. These publications included newsletters, informational pamphlets, and brochures distributed by RESOLVE and other related nonprofit organizations, informational pamphlets and brochures distributed by pharmaceutical companies, literature distributed at the adoption symposium, and RESOLVE's book, *Resolving Infertility*.

I also consulted several of the Centers for Disease Control's ART Reports as well as online and written resources from the American Society for Reproductive Medicine, IVF.com, and Atlanta-area clinics. These written texts (paper and online) provided additional material for a close reading of RESOLVE and the infertility industry to which it is connected.

All of the institutional ephemera used in this book—including local and national RESOLVE newsletters published during 2000–2001, informational pamphlets and patient education booklets distributed by RESOLVE, pamphlets and brochures distributed by pharmaceutical companies, literature distributed at the adoption symposium, RESOLVE fact sheets (for example, on donor eggs), and other such written materials—are in the possession of the author. Readers interested in obtaining copies of documents for review may contact the author directly by writing to Karey Harwood, Department of Philosophy and Religion, Campus Box 8103, North Carolina State University, Raleigh, NC 27695.

Why Use These Methods in an Ethics Book?

In retrospect, one methodological commitment was probably paramount above all others in this book: I had to be open to changing my mind, to letting my observations affect my agenda and take it in new directions. I even had to be open to the fact that what concerned me most at the outset would not seem at all relevant by the end of my yearlong immersion in the infertile world.

I had concerns about ART, about the way it was used, and about what that use said about American society. All of these concerns were rooted in normative values about what is fair, healthy, and good. Yet to proceed with a normative argument about why ART should be curtailed based on my interpretation of a few cultural trends seemed an irresponsible way to "do" ethics. Without firsthand experience with infertility, I felt it was too easy to judge the actions of others and build a generalized argument that avoided the messy, complicating aspects of lived experience. I therefore endeavored to build normative arguments not on speculation, fear, and prejudgments but on concrete realities and complex persons. The particular kind of qualitative research I did also reveals a commitment to the idea that moral decision making is socially shaped, not sprung from isolated acts of abstract deliberation.

My original concerns about gender justice were not ultimately lost but became more complex with details from a social world. These details pertained to why people actually use ART and what seems to be the actual goods and harms that ART enables. These details brought into clearer focus the influence of consumerism and illuminated the meaning making that takes place on the ground, including how people struggle with the meaning that should be given to biological connections with one's child. The research I conducted was itself an important learning process, which I think not only justifies why ethics needs the social sciences but in so doing models a responsible way to do ethics.

Interview Schedule

These questions were designed as open-ended inquiries into the experience of infertility and the values informing individual women's responses to infertility, including the decision to try assisted reproductive technologies (ART). I asked about women's valuing of childbearing generally, some of the factors influencing the decision to have children, how the interviewees approached this decision with their husbands/partners, and some other basic background questions. I sought to set the decision to use ART in the wider context of my interviewee's life and value system.

In addition to investigating personal stories, I probed for a larger perspective on ART and thus asked directly for an opinion about ART's impact on society and on women. I intended to assess individuals' level of interest in connecting their personal experience with larger social issues, such as the issue of delayed childbearing, work and family conflicts, and fair access to infertility treatments. I also attempted to ascertain the various influences on individual decision making. As part of this agenda, I asked questions about the treatment process itself, subjects' interactions with physicians and nurses, and subjects' support systems during treatment.

Since it was apparent from the early stages of my participant observation that infertility is often described as a life-shaping event, I pursued that theme more deeply in the individual interviews. Here I sought to discover how values might have changed, under what influences, and to what end.

I interviewed one male subject, a therapist who had been a discussion leader at a RESOLVE meeting and who had been through the experience of infertility with his wife. All of my other subjects were women who were either currently dealing with infertility or who had resolved their infertility within the previous ten years.

The interviews were semistructured, which means I asked everyone the same basic set of questions listed here but followed my subjects' lead in discussing matters of importance to them.

1. Could you tell me about the circumstances surrounding your discovery of a fertility problem?

a. Duration—when/how did you first find out about the problem you are having?

b. Diagnosis—have your doctors been able to arrive at a diagnosis for the problem?

c. Treatment plan—what is your current approach to addressing the problem?

2. Before your discovery of a fertility problem, could you tell me how you arrived at the decision to have children?

   a. What factors influenced your decision to have children?

   b. If you have a partner, did you and your partner agree/disagree about the importance of having children and about the timing of childbearing?

   c. What would/does being a mother/parent mean to you?

3. Can you walk me through the steps of how you came to the decision to seek treatment for infertility?

   a. What factors were important in the decision?

   b. What resources seemed immediately attractive to you and why?

   c. What avenues for resolving your infertility have opened up for you during the course of your treatment?

   d. What avenues are you unable to consider and why?

   e. What kind of limits have you set (time, financial) for treatment, and why?

4. Tell me about whether you are considering/have considered other ways to build your family.

   a. What factors made you consider/not consider adoption?

   b. What priority do you give adoption with relation to conceiving through assisted reproductive technology or to not having children?

5. Could you describe your support system for dealing with infertility?

   a. What kinds of support have the doctors/nurses provided throughout this process?

   b. Why have you/have you not sought the support of RESOLVE?

   c. What kinds of support has RESOLVE provided?

   d. What were the most helpful meetings or speakers?

   e. How have friends and family reacted?

6. How has this experience changed you?

   a. How has it affected your views about yourself and/or your marriage?

   b. How has it affected your views about being a parent/mother?

   c. How does it differ from other problems you have faced in your life?

   d. What, if anything, about this experience makes you angry? Why?

   e. Knowing what you know now, is there anything you would do differently?

7. In your opinion, what do you think the impact of assisted reproductive technologies has been on society?

   a. What is your opinion about the importance of insurance coverage for infertility treatments?

   b. What is your opinion about the importance of access to infertility treatments?

   c. In what ways do you think assisted reproductive technologies have been beneficial and/or harmful for women?

8. How would you describe yourself and your background?

a. What is your age, marital status, length of marriage?
b. What is your primary occupation? Educational background?
c. If you have a partner, what is his/her primary occupation?
d. What is your religious background?
e. Do you have a religious affiliation currently?
f. Where do you consider yourself to be from?

Notes

Introduction

1. Interview by author, February 26, 2001. Sarah is not the interviewee's real name.

2. Vallis, "McGill Pill Could Reshape Fertility." After leaving McGill, Dr. Roger Gosden served as the scientific director of the Jones Institute for Reproductive Medicine in Norfolk, Virginia, where he pursued efforts to "bank" or freeze ovaries for cancer patients who must undergo chemotherapy. In 2002, Gosden was reported as saying that the technique of ovary freezing, when perfected, would benefit healthy women who elected to store one of their ovaries for use later in life (Connor, "Frozen Ovary Banks"). As of June 2006, he worked at the Center for Reproductive Medicine and Infertility on Manhattan's Upper East Side.

3. There is an obvious difference between the career pill and the constellation of procedures known as ART: ART is aimed exclusively at the achievement of pregnancy, whereas the career pill is envisioned first as a contraceptive but with the benefit of making the achievement of pregnancy possible later in life. ART treats infertility, whereas the career pill would prevent it, but both biotechnologies expand (at least theoretically) the window of opportunity for pregnancy.

4. The constraints of balancing work and family are a burden that falls on families as a whole, especially children. However, a technology such as the career pill underscores the common perception that women are primarily responsible for—and can most easily accommodate—the juggling of childbearing with other life commitments and responsibilities.

5. Folbre, *Invisible Heart*. Crittenden, an economic journalist, makes a very similar argument in *Price of Motherhood*.

6. Chandra and Mosher, "Demography of Infertility." See also Stephen, "Projections of Impaired Fecundity"; Stephen and Chandra, "Use of Infertility Services."

7. Both ART and the career pill make it possible (or may someday make it possible, in the case of the career pill) to extend fertility for women past the biological "norm,"

which is thought to be the twenties and early thirties. However, ART is most successful when it is used to treat infertility in younger women. Success rates decrease significantly for women over forty, which suggests that ART is not in fact an effective remedy for delayed childbearing.

8. See Hewlett, *Creating a Life*, 205.

9. Kalb, "Truth about Fertility." The American Society of Reproductive Medicine, a medical society representing physicians who treat infertility, was apparently responding to a lack of awareness on the part of patients about the role of age in infertility as well as an unjustified confidence about the success of ART for women older than forty. It is an open question whether ASRM accurately interpreted women's understanding of the impact of age on their fertility.

10. I use or at least am inspired by the extended case method as described by Burawoy, *Ethnography Unbound*. The extended case method takes theoretical generalizations and tests/revises them based on qualitative empirical data collected through participant observation.

11. Flyvbjerg, *Making Social Science Matter*, 83.

12. Abu-Lughod, "Writing against Culture," 156. Abu-Lughod defends a research method she calls "ethnographies of the particular," which avoids generalization and gets as close as possible to people's everyday lives as a means of writing "about lives so as to constitute others as less other."

13. Hewlett, *Creating a Life*, 82. Hewlett is quoting one of the women she interviewed from the "breakthrough generation"—women who came of age on the crest of the women's movement and established themselves in careers newly open to women in the 1970s and 1980s. She presents their stories and the wisdom of their experience as a "gift" from one generation of women to the next.

14. Ibid., 281–85.

15. Paying attention to individual stories and individual decision making about infertility is for me a methodological, not ideological, commitment. The value of listening to individual stories lies not, as Hewlett seems to suggest, in discovering new strategies to "beat the system" or "have it all" but in learning what generalizations about ART have missed. I do not view individuals as being able to act apart from or outside of social influences, as free agents without connections to others (that is, I do not embrace an ideology of individualism). Rather, paying attention to particularity is helpful methodologically because it can demonstrate how social influences are embodied in everyday life as well as how individuals act in ways that structural arguments may not have predicted.

16. See Niebuhr, *Responsible Self*. Before Niebuhr, the American pragmatists developed the idea of "reflective intelligence," which Dewey, "Need for a Recovery," describes as a process of learning from experience, of altering knowledge already in one's possession based on experience and creating something novel. Learning is a dynamic function that engages the environment in ways that can fundamentally change the

learner. Learning requires social communication and participation. I believe a natural resonance exists between Dewey's beliefs and Niebuhr's responsible ethics, to which I will return in later chapters.

Chapter One

1. Centers for Disease Control and Prevention, American Society for Reproductive Medicine, Society for Assisted Reproductive Technology, and RESOLVE, "1997 Assisted Reproductive Technology Success Rates," 383.

2. The decision to use GIFT or ZIFT rather than IVF involves a variety of factors. However, the vast majority of ART cycles use IVF. According to Centers for Disease Control and Prevention, American Society for Reproductive Medicine, Society for Assisted Reproductive Technology, and RESOLVE, "1999 Assisted Reproductive Technology Success Rates," for example, 97 percent of ART cycles were IVF, 1 percent were GIFT, 1 percent were ZIFT, and 1 percent were a combination.

3. RESOLVE, with Aronson, *Resolving Infertility*, 178. Cancellation of a cycle of ART occurs in 10–20 percent of cases, according to RESOLVE, "either because a woman has not stimulated well or has overstimulated." Hyperstimulation of the ovaries is a potentially very serious condition. However, neither RESOLVE's *Resolving Infertility* nor the CDC's annual *ART Reports* contains any detailed information about the symptoms of ovarian hyperstimulation syndrome, which in severe cases (1 percent) can cause "blood clots, kidney damage, ovarian torsion (twisting), or abdominal and chest fluid collections" (Duke University Medical Center Web site, <http://www.dukehealth.org>, accessed April 16, 2007).

4. For a more historical review of ART procedures, including the introduction of ICSI in the 1990s, see Hodder, "New Fertility."

5. Institute for Reproductive Medicine at Saint Barnabas Medical Center, "Statement in Regard to Cytoplasmic Transfer."

6. President's Council on Bioethics, *Reproduction and Responsibility*, 62. The Jones Institute in Norfolk, Virginia, was also among the first U.S. clinics to attempt cytoplasmic transfer. The FDA justified the imposition of the Investigational New Drug process on the grounds that cytoplasmic transfer is a form of gene-transfer research because mitochondrial DNA are transferred from one human egg to the other.

7. Stephen and Chandra, "Use of Infertility Services," 132.

8. Centers for Disease Control and Prevention, American Society for Reproductive Medicine, and Society for Assisted Reproductive Technology, "2002 Assisted Reproductive Technology Success Rates."

9. Ibid. The annual "ART Reports" provide maps showing the concentration of ART clinics in the United States and Puerto Rico.

10. RESOLVE, with Aronson, *Resolving Infertility*, 3. The terms "infertility," "fertility problems," and "impaired fecundity" have distinct meanings, which makes a

difference in reporting statistics but which does not have a significant impact on this discussion. To meet the definition of "infertility," a couple would have to be unable to conceive for a period of twelve months.

11. Stephen and Chandra, "Use of Infertility Services," 136.

12. Chandra and Stephen, "Impaired Fecundity," 34.

13. Stephen and Chandra, "Use of Infertility Services," 134.

14. Ibid.

15. Ibid., 136.

16. Ibid. However, I have read some conflicting interpretations of the significance of race with regard to ART use. Some authors claim that blacks make up a disproportionately large percentage of the infertile population. See, for example, Roberts, *Killing the Black Body*, 251. Yet Stephen and Chandra, "Use of Infertility Services," maintain, based on the National Survey of Family Growth data, that infertility similarly affects women of all races and socioeconomic groups, although the races differ in their use of infertility services. Moreover, Stephen and Chandra suggest that socioeconomic status is more determinative of ART use than race. They believe that an unmet need for services exists, particularly among women who are less educated and have less income.

17. Ibid. See also Wilcox and Mosher, "Use of Infertility Services."

18. American Society for Reproductive Medicine Web site.

19. Neumann, Gharib, and Weinstein, "Cost of a Successful Delivery."

20. American Society for Reproductive Medicine, Ethics Committee, "Shared-Risk or Refund Programs."

21. Centers for Disease Control and Prevention, American Society for Reproductive Medicine, Society for Assisted Reproductive Technology, and RESOLVE, "1999 Assisted Reproductive Technology Success Rates."

22. Centers for Disease Control and Prevention, American Society for Reproductive Medicine, and Society for Assisted Reproductive Technology, "2002 Assisted Reproductive Technology Success Rates." For comparison, the 1999 report states that 68.7 percent of ART cycles using fresh, nondonor eggs or embryos did not produce a pregnancy, 30.6 percent produced pregnancies, and 0.7 percent produced ectopic pregnancies. Of those cycles that did produce a pregnancy, 19.2 percent resulted in live single births and 11.4 percent resulted in multiple births (Centers for Disease Control and Prevention, American Society for Reproductive Medicine, Society for Assisted Reproductive Technology, and RESOLVE, "1999 Assisted Reproductive Technology Success Rates").

23. Of the viable pregnancies in 1999, 52.3 percent were singleton pregnancies and 30.2 percent were multiple pregnancies; 14.5 percent resulted in miscarriage; 1.2 percent ended in induced abortion; 1.1 percent had unknown outcomes; and 0.7 percent resulted in stillbirths (Centers for Disease Control and Prevention, American Society for Reproductive Medicine, Society for Assisted Reproductive Technology, and RESOLVE, "1999 Assisted Reproductive Technology Success Rates").

24. Centers for Disease Control and Prevention, American Society for Reproductive Medicine, and Society for Assisted Reproductive Technology, "2002 Assisted Reproductive Technology Success Rates."

25. Ibid.

26. Stephen and Chandra, "Use of Infertility Services," 133–34.

27. Kalb, "Truth about Fertility," 42. See also Massey, "Low Ovarian Reserve."

28. Centers for Disease Control and Prevention, American Society for Reproductive Medicine, and Society for Assisted Reproductive Technology, "2002 Assisted Reproductive Technology Success Rates."

29. Ibid.

30. President's Council on Bioethics, *Reproduction and Responsibility*, 153.

31. I address the relationship of the normative to the descriptive more thoroughly in appendix A.

32. See, for example, Elliot, *Better Than Well*; Engelhardt, *Foundations of Bioethics*; Curlin and Hall, "Red Medicine, Blue Medicine."

33. For an exploration of procreative liberty as it relates to homosexuality, see Murphy, "Should Lesbians Count as Infertile Couples?"

34. Tucker, "Freezing Human Eggs."

35. An objection to egg freezing also appeared in Toner, "Your Medical Questions Answered," 7. Toner writes with regard to using egg freezing as a means to extend fertility, "Egg freezing remains a highly experimental therapy. . . . Whether birth defects are more likely to occur is completely unknown. Until more work is done, patients should not hold out false hope for this method of preserving fertility potential." The implication of his remarks is that harm to children should be weighed against the benefits of preserving fertility potential, whatever those benefits might be.

36. Shklar, *Faces of Injustice*, 66.

37. Spain and Bianchi, *Balancing Act*.

38. Arendell, *Mothering and Motherhood*, compares past and present employment rates: "Racial-ethnic, immigrant, and poor women have combined employment and child raising at relatively high rates across the decades. For instance, Black women's labor participation was nearly 48 percent in 1970, White women's nearly 41 percent, Hispanic women's 39 percent. These proportions increased across all groups so that in 1998, roughly 60 percent of Black women, 58 percent of White women, and 63 percent of Hispanic women (all aged 20 and over) were employed." Arendell cites figures from the U.S. Bureau of the Census for the Bureau of Labor Statistics.

39. Schor, *Overworked American*, 30.

40. Hochschild, *Second Shift*.

41. Jacobs and Gerson, "Who Are the Overworked Americans?"

42. Goodman, "Overwork Overwhelms Families."

43. For a discussion of the ideology of "intensive mothering" and its conflict with the values of the work world, see Hays, *Cultural Contradictions*.

44. Keller, "Dual Earners."

45. Arendell, *Mothering and Motherhood*.

46. Stolberg, "Buying Years." More recently, Jane Swift, the thirty-seven-year-old Republican governor of Massachusetts, elected in 2001, received a lot of media attention because she was pregnant with twins while holding office. One journalist noted that by having her children soon after being elected, she challenged the norm that professional women should wait to have babies until the "professional home stretch." See Bazelton, "See Jane."

47. ART was offered in the United States by 1983. Feminist responses followed shortly thereafter.

48. See, for example, Corea, *Mother Machine*; Spallone, *Beyond Conception*.

49. Ryan, "Justice and Artificial Reproduction," 14, uses the terminology "radical non-interventionist," "moderate interventionist," and "radical interventionist." Ryan notes that these categories were originally proposed by Donchin in "Future of Mothering."

50. Donchin, "Feminist Critiques," 479.

51. Rowland, *Living Laboratories*, 278.

52. Firestone, *Dialectic of Sex*.

53. Ryan, "Justice and Artificial Reproduction," 125.

54. Andrews, "My Body, My Property."

55. Donchin, "Feminist Critiques," 481.

56. Ibid.

57. Ibid., 488.

58. Ibid., 483.

59. For a very helpful overview of feminist scholarship on reproductive technologies in the 1980s as well as the 1990s, see Thompson, "Fertile Ground."

60. Nussbaum, *Sex and Social Justice*, 58. Categorizing Nussbaum as simply "liberal" misses some of the nuance that is the fruit of the exchange between liberalism and communitarianism that has occurred at least since the publication of Rawls's *Political Liberalism* (1993).

61. Ryan, "Justice and Artificial Reproduction," 130.

62. Ibid., 125–26.

63. Ibid., 111.

64. Woliver, "Reproductive Technologies."

65. Feminism perennially wrestles with the question of how to simultaneously advocate "women's well-being" yet avoid oversimplifying or overgeneralizing about what helps or harms women. Which women, under what circumstances? These specific questions must be asked at every opportunity to guard against essentializing, which is one reason why paying attention to the particularities of ART use is so important.

66. Roberts, *Killing the Black Body*, 292.

67. Ibid.

68. Woliver, "Deflective Power."

69. *Eisenstadt v. Baird*, 92 S. Ct. 1029 (1972).

70. *Planned Parenthood v. Casey*, 112 S. Ct. 2791 (1992).

71. Robertson, *Children of Choice*, 39.

72. The areas where Robertson is willing to limit procreative liberty are in non-therapeutic enhancement of offspring, intentional diminishment of offspring, and cloning. He argues that these uses of technology deviate too far from the "core values" of the reproductive experience and what makes it meaningful. He also argues that procreative liberty does not protect behavior during pregnancy and after birth (since women are, after all, "free" to avoid or discontinue a pregnancy), and he therefore argues in favor of some forced interventions in pregnancy. These are strange and paradoxical arguments, given his strenuous defense of liberty interests and equally strenuous attack on the relevance of symbolic meanings.

73. Dworkin, *Life's Dominion*.

74. Robertson, *Children of Choice*, 39.

75. Ibid., 143.

76. See, for example, Paul VI, *Humanae Vitae*; Congregation for the Doctrine of the Faith, "*Donum Vitae*." The prohibition applies to contraception as well as ART. The "inseparability thesis" holds that sex should be tied to reproduction and reproduction should be tied to sex.

77. O'Donovan, *Begotten or Made?*

78. O'Donovan's argument, like that of any ethicist working out of a religious tradition, depends on his interpretation of the values of his tradition. He raises questions of virtue—how the use of assisted reproduction impacts the character of the agents acting—that make sense within the context of his tradition. He questions how ART affects the prospective parents who use it, their marriage relationship, and their respective relationships with the resultant child, and his answers are driven by prior expectations about what is a good parent, a good marriage, and a good person. As I have suggested, religious ethics does not differ from secular modes of inquiry in approaching problems with prior conceptions of the good, which makes it no more or less legitimate to consider the perspective of someone like O'Donovan, who self-identifies as a Christian, than anyone else.

79. Behind O'Donovan's work are the ideas of Jewish philosopher Martin Buber; see Buber, *I and Thou*.

80. More recently, Meilaender, "Child of One's Own," has argued that some uses of ART (for example, embryo grading and selection) can school us to accept a "quality control" approach to having children.

81. See Lebacqz, "Diversity, Disability, and Designer Genes."

82. Cahill, *Sex, Gender, and Christian Ethics*, 218.

83. Cahill shares with Nussbaum a confidence in finding universalizable norms as well as a respect for particularity and difference.

84. Cahill is self-consciously aware of the contentiousness surrounding religion and public reason and thus makes this awareness an explicit part of her discussion and justification of a revised natural-law-inspired ethic. Like O'Donovan, Cahill confesses her faith commitments, but she believes she can give reasons that are more publicly accessible.

85. Cahill's chapter on the birth technologies compares and critiques three public documents for their moral arguments about assisted reproduction: the Congregation for the Doctrine of the Faith's *"Donum Vitae"* (1987), the United Kingdom Committee of Inquiry into Human Fertilisation and Embryology's *Report* (1984), and the U.S. Congress, Office of Technology Assessment's *Infertility* (1988).

86. One problem with third-party donors is that this technique opens the door to the logical extreme of collaborative reproduction: see, for example, *In re Marriage of Buzzanca*, 61 Cal. App. 4th 1410, 72 Cal. Rptr. 2d 280 (1998). In this case, a couple contracted with an egg donor, a sperm donor, and a surrogate to produce for them a child. However, the couple divorced before the child was born, at which time the husband revived an argument based on biological ties: because he was not genetically related to the child, he should be relieved of his duties of child support. He was not the "father." The court did not accept his argument, deciding instead that the people who intended the birth of this child are her parents.

87. Cahill, *Sex, Gender, and Christian Ethics*, 254.

88. Cahill is a strong supporter of adoption and has adopted children of her own.

89. While some argue that ART emphasizes social parenthood over biological parenthood and that this is a good, others point out that ART can emphasize the exact reverse: a biological, genetic tie to at least one parent becomes more important than no biological tie at all, as in adoption. A major ethical issue that does not receive attention here is the use of ART by homosexual couples. ART clearly expands the options for creating families and thus radically challenges some dominant cultural views about what counts as a family.

90. Cahill, *Sex, Gender, and Christian Ethics*, 218.

91. Ibid., 55.

92. Berg, "Listening to the Voices," 80.

Chapter Two

1. See appendix A for meeting topics.

2. The hormone human chorionic gonadotrophin, which passes into maternal circulation, is produced only by the human embryo. It is thus a useful indicator of pregnancy during the first eight weeks.

3. Intrauterine insemination is a procedure in which specially prepared sperm are deposited directly into the uterus at the time of ovulation. IVF generally refers to a procedure in which an egg is fertilized in a laboratory dish and the resultant embryo is placed in the woman's uterus.

4. Author's observation, February 3, 2001.

5. Ibid.

6. RESOLVE: The National Infertility Organization, Web site.

7. Ibid.

8. Ibid.

9. RESOLVE: The National Infertility Organization, Web site; RESOLVE and the National Endowment for Financial Education, *Planning to Afford Family Building*.

10. RESOLVE, *Infertility and Insurance Coverage*.

11. RESOLVE, "Advocacy Action" (e-mail update), Spring 2001; Doyle, "Advocacy Action," 12. See also Hidlebaugh, Thompson, and Berger, "Cost of Assisted Reproductive Technologies." Hidlebaugh, Thompson, and Berger conclude that the ART cycle cost per HMO plan member would be $2.49 per annum. There were 295 cycles per million population.

12. Roberts, *Killing the Black Body*, 290. Roberts relies on a 1996 ABC news report.

13. RESOLVE, *Infertility and Insurance Coverage*, 1.

14. RESOLVE, with Aronson, *Resolving Infertility*, 64. More specifically, the causes of infertility include physical blockages (for example, scarred fallopian tubes), hormonal problems (for example, elevated follicle-stimulating hormone, polycystic ovarian syndrome), recurrent miscarriage, problems with sperm count and sperm motility, and many others.

15. These may be weak reasons. A great deal of discussion occurs in the bioethics community about possible birth defects resulting from IVF, cryopreservation of embryos, and the intracytoplasmic sperm injection technique. Studies on the long-term effects of IVF have had great difficulty obtaining funding (group e-mail exchange on the Feminist Approaches to Bioethics listserv, November 18, 2002, posting from Glenn McGee, University of Pennsylvania, editor in chief, *American Journal of Bioethics*).

16. *RESOLVE of Georgia Newsletter*, Summer 2001, 12.

17. See RESOLVE and the National Partnership for Women and Families, *Infertility and Adoption*; National Partnership for Women and Families, *Guide to the Family and Medical Leave Act*.

18. Pappert, "Special Report," 47–48.

19. President's Council on Bioethics, *Reproduction and Responsibility*, 47–51.

20. Ibid., 64–65.

21. Ibid., 51–55.

22. Center for Drug Evaluation and Research, New and Generic Drug Approvals: 1998–2004.

23. President's Council on Bioethics, *Reproduction and Responsibility*, 55–63.

24. RESOLVE, "Overview."

25. Diane Clapp, e-mail to author, July 3, 2005.

26. In a letter from its board of directors and director of government affairs, RESOLVE complained to the President's Council on Bioethics, which would like to

collect and publish more data on ART, that the 1992 law already compiles adequate data and in fact was reporting data that restricted patient freedom of choice and access to services. The letter claimed that the current reporting system "had in some cases had the effect of hurting patients who were denied treatment because their lowered chance of having a baby dissuaded clinics from treating them and risking their statistics" (Lee Collins and Erin Kramer to Leon Kass, December 16, 2003, available at <www.resolve.org>, accessed December 2004).

27. Interview by author, May 25, 2001. There is a nascent literature connecting ovarian cancer and ART.

28. On one occasion, separate discussion groups were held for men and women.

29. Interview by author, January 25, 2001.

30. This statement appears in identical form in a variety of RESOLVE publications and on the group's local and national Web sites.

31. There are many plausible reasons why the number of people in RESOLVE who are living child-free was relatively low, just as there may be many reasons why no one in the group used surrogacy. My observations found that the participants at the monthly meetings had some palpable discomfort with the child-free option. With the exception of one outspoken therapist who often addressed the group and made every effort to convey the message that her life was happy and healthy, many members approached the child-free option as representing defeat. One child-free woman who spoke at a meeting cried during her presentation and did not convey the sense that she had fully resolved her infertility. Far fewer clues explain why surrogacy was rare. The primary reason may be simply that it is prohibitively expensive and more difficult to arrange, plus the woman loses out on the deeply valued experience of pregnancy and childbirth.

32. In brief, shared-risk programs are a way to reduce the financial risk of undergoing several rounds of IVF. After a very careful physical screening for participation in the program, the patient / customer pays a set fee for a certain number of IVF cycles. If the patient conceives during the first cycle, she will have overpaid. But if all of the allotted IVF cycles fail, the patient is shielded from losing thousands of dollars.

33. Aronson, "Value of a Non-Profit," 3.

34. Rausch, "Trust," 1.

35. Cook, "Religion and Infertility."

36. The May 2000 meeting was called "Life after Infertility: Pregnancy after Infertility, Parenting after Infertility, and Childfree Living."

37. Weschler, *Taking Charge of Your Fertility*, 342–43.

38. See Starr, *Social Transformation*; Sherwin, *No Longer Patient*; Morgen, *Into Our Own Hands*.

39. RESOLVE's membership includes both women and men, and all the meetings I attended included both women and men. RESOLVE also has a more respectful attitude toward the medical profession. While RESOLVE uses all the politically correct medical terms and seeks to empower infertility patients, it does not, as an organization,

share with the Boston Women's Health Book Collective or with the Feminist International Network of Resistance to Reproductive and Genetic Engineering a deep suspicion of the medical establishment.

40. Ruzek, "History and Future."

41. RESOLVE Corporate Council Web site.

42. See van Balen, "Psychologization of Infertility."

43. RESOLVE, *When You're Wishing for a Baby*. This informational pamphlet is aimed primarily at establishing infertility as a legitimate medical condition. One example of the myths/facts discussed is, "Myth: It's all in your head! Why don't you relax and take a vacation. Then you'll get pregnant. Fact: Infertility is a disease or condition of the reproductive system. While relaxing may help you with your overall quality of life, the stress and deep emotions you feel are the result of infertility, not the cause of it."

44. Sandelowski and de Lacy, "Uses of a 'Disease.'"

45. Beck, "Making the Leap," 6.

46. Ibid.

47. Ibid., 7.

48. Swidler, "In Groups We Trust."

49. Wuthnow, *Sharing the Journey*, 340.

50. RESOLVE uses the metaphor of the journey with considerable frequency. See, for example, RESOLVE with Aronson, *Resolving Infertility*, part 2 of which is titled "The Medical Journey."

51. One woman I interviewed, for example, described being continually questioned by another support group member about the outcome of every IVF cycle. She felt the woman's inquisitiveness was based less on concern for her well-being and more on individual competitiveness: who could achieve pregnancy first. By contrast, she described the RESOLVE monthly meetings as a place where she went to "sit there and learn" (interview by author, September 11, 2001).

52. See Heatherley, *Balcony People*.

53. Wuthnow, *Sharing the Journey*, 201.

54. See Fraser, "Rethinking the Public Sphere."

55. Eliasoph, *Avoiding Politics*.

56. Wuthnow, *Sharing the Journey*, 187.

Chapter Three

1. Author's observation, January 2, February 6, 2001.

2. Author's observation, February 6, 2001.

3. For a thorough account of the diverse racial, ethnic, religious, and socioeconomic contexts that differently affect the experiences of American women using reproductive technologies (particularly prenatal testing), see Rapp, *Testing Women*. Although confined to one major metropolitan area, New York City, Rapp's anthropological research

brought her into contact with a tremendous range of individuals considering amnio-centesis and thus illuminated much greater diversity than can be demonstrated here with regard to varied cultural norms.

4. Author's observation, January 2, 2001.

5. Author's observation, November 21, 2000.

6. Ibid.

7. One couple with secondary infertility attended regularly throughout the year I observed, and they seemed to be accepted by other group members. People with primary and secondary infertility are separated for the therapist-led living room support groups.

8. Author's observation, December 5, 2000.

9. Ibid.

10. Author's observation, March 20, 2001.

11. Author's observation, October 10, 2000, January 2, 2001.

12. Interview by author, January 25, 2001.

13. Author's observation, January 2, 2001.

14. Evidence-based medicine is simply collating data from many different empirical studies to find out whether a certain treatment works. It is contrasted with the practice of prescribing medical treatments based on long-standing tradition or custom.

15. Author's observation, January 2, 2001.

16. Author's observation, December 5, 2000.

17. Ibid.

18. E-mail to author, March 8, 2001.

19. Interview by author, March 1, 2001.

20. Interview by author, February 26, 2001.

21. <www.IVF.com> chat room, January 10, 2001.

22. Clinics also vary with regard to the number of embryos they are willing to implant in any given IVF cycle. More responsible clinics limit the number of embryos to two or three to avoid the possibility of a high-order multiple gestation. Other clinics, often simply following the patient's desire to keep costs down, implant four or more embryos at once to increase the odds of achieving a pregnancy.

23. Author's observation, February 3, 2001.

24. Author's observation, December 5, 2000.

25. Interview by author, February 26, 2001.

26. Ibid.

27. Interview by author, February 28, 2001.

28. Author's observation, February 3, March 20, 2001. Participants frequently used the phrase "treadmill of infertility" to refer to the treatment process.

29. No meetings dealt with the particular issues experienced by homosexual couples who desire to conceive children. The group's general stance against moralizing would

probably lead members to accept a homosexual couple in their midst. The occasion never arose to test this hypothesis, however.

30. Lasker and Borg, *In Search of Parenthood*.

31. Author's observation, December 5, 2000.

32. Author's observation, February 6, 2001.

33. Author's observation, March 20, 2001.

34. Interview by author, May 25, 2001.

35. Interview by author, March 1, 2001.

36. Author's observation, February 6, 2001.

37. Interview by author, February 28, 2001.

38. Ibid.

39. Author's observation, February 3, 2001.

40. Author's observation, March 20, 2001.

41. Clements, "Process of Understanding."

42. Interview by author, February 15, 2001.

43. Author's observation, January 2, 2001.

44. Interview by author, January 25, 2001.

45. Author's observation, January 2, 2001.

46. Ibid.

47. Author's observation, December 5, 2000.

48. Author's observation, February 3, 2001.

49. Author's observation, October 10, 2000.

50. Author's observation, November 21, 2000.

51. Author's observation, January 2, 2001.

52. Interview by author, March 1, 2001.

53. Author's observation, February 3, 2001.

54. Author's observation, April 3, 2001.

55. It was not possible to gain a sense of the financial limitations of every person or couple that attended RESOLVE meetings. One of the copresidents shared her views on the importance of insurance coverage in an interview: "I think, of course, mandated infertility insurance coverage would be wonderful because that way more people could have access to getting treatment. . . . There are so many people that cannot pursue their dreams because they can't afford it. You know, we're talking about eight thousand to twelve thousand dollars per IVF cycle. Egg donors [are] sometimes fifteen thousand dollars. Adoption, depending on what you do, anywhere from twelve thousand dollars to twenty-five thousand or thirty thousand" (interview by author, January 25, 2001).

56. Interview by author, April 8, 2001.

57. Author's observation, February 3, 2001.

58. Interview by author, April 8, 2001.

59. Author's observation, November 21, 2000.

60. Interview by author, April 8, 2001.

61. Kolata, "Fertility, Inc."

62. Author's observation, January 2, 2001.

63. The rest of what he said is as follows: "Ninety percent of the [academic] papers out there are garbage and don't really tell you how to treat patients." Some papers are written solely "to advance up the academic food chain . . . and are so narrowly designed for research purposes, they don't really tell us much" (author's observation, January 2, 2001).

64. Georgia Reproductive Specialists Web site.

65. Interview by author, January 25, 2001; Author's observation, January 2, 2001.

66. Interview by author, February 15, 2001.

67. Interview by author, February 26, 2001.

68. Interview by author, February 28, 2001. Doctors may also become the object of blame (interview by author, March 1, 2001).

69. Interview by author, February 28, 2001.

70. A number of local adoption agencies came to the symposium to advertise their services. Several classrooms in the education building of the church had been converted into informational booths for these agencies. Brightly colored pictures of children's faces were pinned to poster boards propped on tables, which also held stacks of informational pamphlets. Another room housed a sale of books on various aspects of the infertility experience and adoption process. Two examples from the book sale were *Sweet Grapes: How to Stop Being Infertile and Start Living Again*, about the transition from infertility to adoption, and *When Empty Arms Become a Heavy Burden*, about faith issues and infertility.

71. Drawing on Elizabeth Bartholet's argument, Cahill notes that "adoption laws, health insurance policies, and the medicalized infertility scenario conspire to make it easier for parents to seek high-tech therapies than to parent already-existing children" (*Sex, Gender, and Christian Ethics*, 247). Roberts, *Killing the Black Body*, argues that race is a factor motivating the use of egg/sperm donors to have a white child and that race has been a factor in lawsuits over some clinics' mishandling of gametes (when the resulting child was the wrong race).

72. Author's observation, December 5, 2000.

73. See Gudorf, "Parenting, Mutual Love, and Sacrifice."

74. Interview by author, March 1, 2001.

75. Author's observation, November 21, 2000.

76. Interview by author, January 25, 2001.

77. Interview by author, April 8, 2001.

78. Author's observation, December 5, 2000.

79. In an ectopic pregnancy, the embryo implants in a fallopian tube rather than in the uterus. Ectopic pregnancies must be terminated because they endanger the life of the mother and are incompatible with the healthy development of the fetus.

80. Author's observation, November 21, 2000.

81. Interview by author, September 20, 2001.

82. Author's observation, March 20, 2001.

83. Ibid.

84. Ibid.

85. Interview by author, February 26, 2001.

86. Alice Domar, the featured speaker at RESOLVE's April 2001 Mind/Body Women's Retreat, referred to a study of faith and infertility that found that infertility often causes a crisis in faith that can encourage in some people the development of a more sophisticated faith perspective. She referred to "levels" or stages of faith.

87. Interview by author, February 26, 2001.

88. Interview by author, May 25, 2001.

89. For a discussion of the link between secularity and pluralism, see Berger, "From the Crisis of Religion to the Crisis of Secularity."

90. Interview by author, February 28, 2001.

91. Interview by author, March 1, 2001.

92. Interview by author, May 25, 2001.

93. For RESOLVE's official position, see RESOLVE, *Fact Sheet: Donor Egg*, a fascinating and provocative document that describes the history of egg donation and discusses the issue of whether to disclose the use of an egg donor to the resultant child.

94. According to the physician who spoke that night, women who need donated eggs fall into the following categories: menopause/perimenopause ("surprisingly young women sometimes have this condition"); oophorectomy (removal of ovaries); elevated follicle-stimulating hormone regardless of age ("elevated FSH usually closes the door on IVF, or it should"); "low responders" (women who do not respond to the drugs given to stimulate the ovaries); severe polycystic ovarian syndrome; and previously abnormal IVF cycle (the embryo developed abnormally).

95. Author's observation, April 3, 2001. According to the physician who spoke, in 1999, her clinic's "ongoing pregnancy rate" was 45 percent for IVF with donor eggs. In 2000, that rate was 60 percent. This is much higher than the national average for IVF with nondonated eggs.

96. For a fuller discussion of this argument, see Anderson, "Is Women's Labor a Commodity?"

97. Ginsberg and Rapp, *Conceiving the New World Order*, 1–18.

98. During her presentation, the physician said that women of this generation tend to look younger and fitter than their mothers and grandmothers did at the same age. "They work out, look like a million bucks . . . but their reproductive age is still the same or even more advanced."

99. This particular clinic allows women up to forty-eight years old to receive donor eggs. Other programs have age limits in the fifties or no age limit at all, but the physician seemed a little uncomfortable about helping substantially older women be-

come pregnant: "You have to consider the welfare of the child . . . and the health of the parent" (author's observation, April 3, 2001).

100. Ibid.

101. Egg donors can command much higher fees. See Mead, "Eggs for Sale." See also Thomasma, "Selling Human Egg Donation"; Stock, "Eggs for Sale."

102. Author's observation, April 3, 2001.

103. This particular clinic does not allow more than three donations, both because of the risk of cancer to the donor and the risk to the gene pool. Other clinics have other guidelines. Risks to recipients include age-related obstetric risks and the risk of multiple-fetus pregnancy. Physical risks to children are not fully known.

104. Donor selection was also discussed as a process of "matching." The clinic looks for physical characteristics, blood type, and the "must haves" specified by the recipient couple. Blood type is important for keeping the egg donation confidential in the future. To explain what she meant by "must haves," the physician told a story of a patient who came in and said, "I gotta have a Michelle Pfeiffer." The physician was incredulous at first, because some health problems had made this woman a little overweight and puffy in the face. But when the patient brought in a photograph of herself from her mid-twenties (the age of most donors), the physician was amazed: "I'll be darned if she didn't look exactly like Michelle Pfeiffer." To help with the matching of physical characteristics, the clinic asks recipients to bring in a photograph of themselves at the age of the potential donor. In Atlanta, clinics apparently can match physical characteristics with some specificity because many donors exist. In a place such as Ohio, noted the physician, "you can only match by race" because few donors are available.

105. Author's observation, May 15, 2001.

106. Author's observation, April 3, 2001.

107. Interview by author, April 8, 2001.

108. Author's observation, April 3, 2001.

109. Ibid.

110. Ibid.

111. Ibid.

112. Interview by author, February 26, 2001.

113. Interview by author, April 8, 2001.

114. Author's observation, May 15, 2001.

115. I have also referred to this issue as the problem of setting limits. Most limit setting is dictated by financial, medical, and legal considerations, although therapists also discussed emotional limits with the group: it would be time to stop if one is becoming too depressed by the process, for example, or if it is seriously straining the marriage.

Chapter Four

1. The clinic representatives who came to present information about egg and sperm donors and surrogacy seemed especially hopeful that egg donation might someday be as commonplace as sperm donation, which has a longer history and broader use. A representative from a well-established Atlanta sperm bank, Xytex, was present in the audience that night. Like many sperm banks, Xytex allows prospective users to "shop" online for donors according to physical characteristics. The identity of donors is kept confidential, but baby pictures are available for viewing. Unlike the practice of using donated eggs to become pregnant, the use of donated sperm has notably broadened beyond people who are experiencing medical infertility to include single women and lesbian couples.

2. Egg freezing or banking is at the research stage and is just beginning to become available to the public in 2007. Extend Fertility, a company based in Woburn, Massachusetts, now markets egg freezing to women.

3. For example, trying IVF with women who have elevated levels of follicle-stimulating hormone is a controversial decision. Many physicians believe it is futile and irresponsible to try IVF under these circumstances.

4. Author's observation, January 2, 2001.

5. For an excellent overview of feminist critiques of science, technology, and medicine as they relate to reproductive technologies, see Thompson, "Fertile Ground."

6. These differences thus include both biological differences between men and women (who gestate the pregnancy) and more socially constructed differences about the meaning of fertility / infertility and motherhood for women. I do not mean to imply that these differences can be cleanly divided simply into either nature or culture, only that the group constantly interpreted and reinterpreted different kinds of "differences."

7. Interview by author, March 1, 2001.

8. Pollitt, "Backlash Babies."

9. See Miller-McLemore, "Produce or Perish"; Miller-McLemore, *Also a Mother*.

10. Miller-McLemore, "Produce or Perish," 56.

11. I appreciate the voices within feminism that have reevaluated motherhood and resisted the tendency to equate it with women's oppression. For example, scholars such as Glendon have criticized liberal feminism for replicating the dominant culture's disregard for unpaid "care work," assuming that only paid employment "counts" toward sexual equality, and for dismissing women's desires for family ("Is the Economic Emancipation of Women Today Contrary to a Healthy, Functioning Family?").

12. I owe the idea of ART as ascesis to my colleagues in the Graduate Division of Religion, Emory University, Ethics and Society colloquy, April 3, 2001. I thank especially Ted Smith and Timothy Jackson.

13. See appendix B for interview schedule.

14. Author's observation, April 3, 2001.

15. This rationale would support the future practice of egg freezing / ovary banking.

16. Woliver, "Deflective Power"; Roberts, *Killing the Black Body*, 292.

17. In *Gender Vertigo*, Risman develops Okin's ideas about the structuring effects of gender and how we might move beyond them to build humanist principles of justice.

18. Okin, *Justice, Gender, and the Family*.

19. Kittay, *Love's Labor*.

20. Folbre, *Invisible Heart*.

21. Benhabib, *Situating the Self*, 77–78.

22. Shklar, *Faces of Injustice*, distinguishes between injustice and misfortune, reminding us that we need not accept seemingly natural phenomena (for example, women's more limited time frame for biological reproduction) as "misfortune." How we respond to "natural" phenomena advances or undermines justice. Justice is a human ideal, and the structures of society that support or undermine it are human constructs.

23. In *Barren in the Promised Land*, May discusses the history of infertility and how it has in modern times been constructed as an illness needing medical treatment.

24. Author's observation, April 7, 2001.

25. Some of the RESOLVE leaders who attended the retreat seemed displeased with Domar's comments that women trying to become pregnant should ease up on exercise and not worry too much about gaining weight. Apparently, many of them used exercise as a way to cope with the stress of infertility treatments, which they explained in small-group discussions when Domar was not present. In addition to saying it was better to be ten pounds overweight than ten pounds underweight when trying to become pregnant, Domar also openly criticized our culture's obsession with thinness—its message that "being thin is more important than procreating" (author's observation, April 7, 2001).

26. Author's observation, April 7, 2001.

27. Ibid.

28. Ibid.

29. Stephen and Chandra, "Use of Infertility Services," 136.

30. See Roberts, *Killing the Black Body*, 246–93.

31. The copresident I interviewed very clearly stated her support of health insurance coverage in terms of extending access to ART to more people.

32. Schor, "What's Wrong with Consumer Society?" 41.

33. Ibid., 39.

34. Meyer, "Self and Life Course."

35. For example, Cahill, *Sex, Gender, and Christian Ethics*, argues that the infertility industry and the media fuel a climate of desperation and that the "technological imperative" seduces many infertile couples into endless trials of IVF. Meanwhile, unwanted children already in existence go unadopted. She contends that the infertility industry plays on infertile couples' sense of inadequacy and the all-too-American need to buy something to fix a problem.

36. Schor, *Overworked American*, 120.

37. Rosenblatt, *Consuming Desires*, 19.

38. When I interviewed the therapist who told the RESOLVE group members that they did not need to feel as though they had to "keep up with the Joneses," she explained that competitiveness was not so much the issue as an overwhelming feeling of inadequacy, accompanied by a need to try everything possible to avoid regret (interview by author, May 25, 2001).

39. Author's observation, February 3, 2001.

40. Rosenblatt, *Consuming Desires*, 18.

41. Cahill, *Sex, Gender, and Christian Ethics*, 218.

42. Kurzman, "Convincing Sociologists."

43. Ibid., 251. He was evaluating the ethnographic projects of his classmates in this article.

44. See Taylor, "All-Consuming Experience."

45. Author's observation, January 2, 2001.

46. Ibid.

47. The normative position I have in mind is one that believes almost everything can have a market value. This value is then weighed against costs to find the utility of a thing, person, idea, or whatever.

48. I draw primarily from Weber, *Protestant Ethic*. In this and other writings, he elaborates his idea of rationalization, a process of social evolution governed by strategic instrumental reason. We end up in the iron cage, in part, because the "How shall we live?" questions—which are the kinds of questions asked by religion—fall outside the rational. They are about normative values.

49. Habermas incorporates Hegel's critiques of Kant. The intersubjectivity in Habermas's discourse ethics is a major point of difference from Rawls's hypothetical and individualistic original position.

50. Cahill, *Sex, Gender, and Christian Ethics*, 46.

51. Both Cahill and Nussbaum want to avoid what they interpret as the relativistic implications of postmodernism because, they argue, relativism can enervate forceful moral critique across different cultures and within pluralistic cultures such as the United States.

52. Nussbaum, *Sex and Social Justice*, 41. Her list includes life; bodily health and integrity; senses, imagination, thought; emotions; practical reason; affiliation; other species; play; and control over one's environment, both political and material.

53. Nussbaum, *Sex and Social Justice*, carefully explains her relationship to the liberal tradition (which she derives selectively through Kant, Mill, and Aristotle), why women need more individualism rather than less, and why freedom and choice are so important. She wants to preserve maximum freedom to pursue individual life plans while ensuring that certain structures and safeguards are in place to make the realistic exercise of freedom possible.

54. I do not believe that RESOLVE members were brazen libertarians. Nothing in my research would support this conclusion. Rather, they are wounded and resentful of their situation, which they believe is unfair. The "liberty" to use ART—such as it is, for those who can afford it—only partially mitigates this deeper sense of being wronged by infertility. It is important not to lose sight of the human reality in considering abstract arguments about procreative liberty.

55. This phrase comes from Robertson, *Children of Choice*, which is considered his major work on the subject and represents a comprehensive examination of different types of assisted reproduction (for example, artificial insemination, IVF, and surrogacy) as well as the issues of contraception, abortion, and nonreproductive uses of reproductive capacities (for example, research on embryos).

56. See, for example, Ryan, "Argument for Unlimited Procreative Liberty."

57. Glendon discusses how traditional American ideas about property were "welded . . . to certain of J. S. Mill's enormously influential views about personal liberty" (*Rights Talk*, 52). The phrase "right to be let alone" was coined in Brandeis and Warren, "Right to Privacy."

58. This version of individual liberty (prominent in legal decisions) finds its roots in Mill, although one could argue that it takes the emphasis on individuality and the irreducible value of the individual from Mill's *On Liberty* (1859) without also incorporating Mill's attention to the social dimensions of individual freedom.

59. Feminists have long criticized the public/private split that runs through social contract theory and pervasively influences ideas about autonomy and freedom. These critiques generally highlight the missing dimension of sociality—for example, how the "background" care work typically done by women was taken for granted and how human beings were assumed to be more atomistic and self-sustaining than is realistic.

60. *Casey v. Planned Parenthood*, 112 S. Ct. 2791 (1992).

61. *Bragdon v. Abbott*, 66 U.S.L.W. 4601 (June 26, 1998).

62. Wolf, "Pre-Implantation Genetic Diagnosis." Wolf argues that reproductive medicine requires a special ethics. The decision making is never only about the present, the people who can talk, but is oriented toward the future. No one would use this medicine without the desire for a baby. It is important to balance parental wishes with the potential child's well-being in a context of increasing parental desperation. She says that in her experience with IVF, she drew the line at cytoplasmic transfer and did so on behalf of her wanted child. There are no animal studies of cytoplasmic transfer: human beings are the experiment.

63. Bellah et al., *Good Society*, 286. See also Madsen et al., *Meaning and Modernity*.

64. Bellah et al., *Good Society*, 286.

65. Ibid., 287–89.

66. Ibid., 306.

67. Fraser, "Rethinking the Public Sphere."

68. Aronson, "Value of a Non-Profit."

69. Glenn McGee, e-mail, Feminist Approaches to Bioethics listserv, November 18, 2002.

70. Diethylstilbestrol (DES) was a drug widely used in the 1950s and 1960s to prevent miscarriages that caused reproductive cancer in girls born to mothers who took the drug. ART uses powerful hormones, and the long-term effects for women are not known.

71. Reported by Johns Hopkins Medical Institutes, November 15, 2002: "After studying data from a national registry of patients with Beckwith-Wiedemann syndrome (BWS), the researchers found that IVF-initiated conception was six times more common than in the general population" (press release, available at <www.hopkinsm edicine.org/press/2002/November/021115.htm>, accessed April 24, 2007). See DeBaun, Niemitz, and Feinberg, "Association of in Vitro Fertilization."

72. RESOLVE: The National Infertility Organization, Web site.

73. President's Council on Bioethics, *Reproduction and Responsibility.*

74. Testimony of Suzi Leather before President's Council on Bioethics, October 18, 2002, <http://bioethicsprint.bioethics.gov/transcripts/oct02/session6.html>, accessed November 23, 2004.

75. O'Connor, "U.S. Infant Mortality Rate Rises Slightly."

76. Lee Collins and Erin Kramer to Leon Kass, December 16, 2003, available at <www.resolve.org>, accessed December 2004.

77. Ibid.

Chapter Five

1. Author's observation, December 5, 2000.

2. Ibid.

3. Author's observation, February 6, 2001.

4. Interview by author, February 26, 2001.

5. Author's observation, February 6, 2001.

6. Author's observation, December 5, 2000.

7. Author's observation, February 6, 2001.

8. In a chemical pregnancy, the conceptus is lost very early, even before a gestational sac can be detected on ultrasound.

9. Interview by author, January 25, 2001.

10. Interview by author, February 15, 2001.

11. Author's observation, January 2, 2001.

12. Ibid.

13. As discussed in the previous chapter, there are many physical differences in what women and men experience in the diagnosis/treatment of infertility. However, men were a steady and welcome presence at RESOLVE meetings. All of these men seemed deeply interested in and sympathetic to their wife's/partner's bodily experiences.

14. Cahill, *Sex, Gender, and Christian Ethics*, 217. Although the larger project of Cahill's work involves developing an ethic that is inductive and respectful of concrete and situated persons, Cahill does not look directly at the experience of users of ART. She relies heavily on secondary reporting and the media's construction of a "rhetoric of desperation" about infertility.

15. A common motto on RESOLVE literature is "All babies are precious. RESOLVE babies are the most precious." Why? Perhaps because of how badly they were wanted and the great lengths to which their parents went to have them. A woman I interviewed explained, "I think if it ended up that we had a child, our biological child, that would just be incredible and so much more valuable now because we're very much facing the reality that that may never happen" (interview by author, April 8, 2001).

16. Author's observation, March 20, 2001.

17. Interview by author, January 25, 2001.

18. The presence of lifelong RESOLVE members clearly demonstrated the existence of an important diachronic story that deserved attention. Over time, through dealing with infertility, people's perspectives changed. During interviews, I probed for changing perspectives based on what I heard in the monthly meetings. See appendix B.

19. I owe this insight to a conversation with Steve Tipton.

20. Kübler-Ross, *On Death and Dying*.

21. Author's observation, March 20, 2001.

22. Author's observation, February 6, 2001.

23. Author's observation, February 3, 2001.

24. Author's observation, February 6, 2001.

25. Author's observation, February 3, 2001.

26. Reich, "Speaking of Suffering," 85. Reich draws his typology from Soelle's *Suffering*, particularly her discussion of suffering and language.

27. Reich, "Speaking of Suffering," 86.

28. Ibid., 89–90.

29. In a sharp critique of Hewlett, *Creating a Life*, and the "high-achieving" women Hewlett describes who lament their childlessness, Pollitt quips that for many people these days, " 'have kids' occupies a place on the to-do list somewhere between 'learn Italian' and 'exercise' " ("Backlash Babies"). Has infertility become a particularly bourgeois form of suffering? Contraception, the separation of sex and marriage, and changing ideas about the timetable for children have affected the meaning of infertility, in particular for different socioeconomic classes.

30. Author's observation, January 2, 2001.

31. The original story was written by Emily Perl Kingsley in 1987. There is now a "Welcome to Holland" Web site for parents of children with Down syndrome. See <www.our-kids.org/Archives/Holland.html>, accessed September 2002; <http://www.nas.com/downsyn/>, accessed September 2002.

32. Author's observation, February 3, 2001.

33. Ibid.

34. Ibid.

35. Author's observation, May 16, 2000.

36. Interview by author, February 26, 2001.

37. Ibid.

38. Ibid.

39. Author's observation, September 19, 2000, February 3, 2001. In these meetings, participants very clearly expressed their understanding that infertility led them to adopt the particular children they now call their own. For a poignant personal reflection on this point, see Volf, "Gift of Infertility."

40. Interview by author, January 25, 2001.

41. Interview by author, February 15, 2001.

42. Inhorn, *Local Babies*, 20.

43. Ibid.

44. Ibid.

45. Cook, "Religion and Infertility."

46. Author's observation, February 6, 2001.

47. Author's observation, March 20, 2001.

48. Soelle, *Suffering*, 67–70.

49. Author's observation, February 6, 2001.

50. Interview by author, September 11, 2001.

51. O'Donovan, *Begotten or Made?*

52. See Holland, "Contested Commodities"; Radin, *Contested Commodities*; Mead, "Eggs for Sale."

53. See Parens, "Goodness of Fragility." More recently, Sandel, "Case against Perfection," 52, has written about the importance of parents having an "openness to the unbidden" when they welcome their children. He makes an eloquent, non-religiously-based argument against genetic enhancement.

54. Davis, "Genetic Dilemmas."

55. Author's observation, April 3, 2001.

56. Interview by author, February 26, 2001.

57. Roberts, *Killing the Black Body*, 272.

58. Cahill, *Sex, Gender, and Christian Ethics*, 247.

59. Author's observation, February 6, 2001.

60. Young, *Intersecting Voices*, 106.

61. Cahill, *Sex, Gender, and Christian Ethics*, 252.

62. Ibid., 253.

63. Ibid.

64. In the case of *In re Marriage of Buzzanca*, a child was conceived with donated eggs and sperm and through the services of a surrogate. After the intended parents divorced, the California Supreme Court eventually ruled that the persons who in-

tended for the child to be conceived were her legal parents (*In re Marriage of Buzzanca*, 61 Cal. App. 4th 1410, 72 Cal. Rptr. 2d 280 [1998]).

65. See especially Judith Butler's essay in Benhabib et al., *Feminist Contentions*, 35–57.

66. Author's observation, March 20, 2001.

Conclusion

1. Rapp, *Testing Women*, 306.

2. Weil, "Wrongful Birth?"

3. Spar, *Baby Business*.

4. In "abortion wars," I include everything from pharmacists who refuse to fill legitimate, legal prescriptions for birth control pills or the morning-after pill to the issues of late-term abortions, parental notification for minors seeking abortions, elective abortions following prenatal diagnosis of defect or disability, and so forth.

5. Rosen, *Preaching Eugenics*.

6. Ibid., 150; Oliver Wendell Holmes in *Buck v. Bell*, U.S. 200 (1927).

7. Dewey believes that philosophy should be useful to people and should endeavor to improve the social welfare of human beings. See especially Dewey, "Need for a Recovery."

8. Shklar, *Faces of Injustice*.

Appendix A

1. Flyvbjerg, *Making Social Science Matter*, 79.

2. Burawoy, *Ethnography Unbound*, 281.

3. Emerson, Fretz, and Shaw, *Writing Ethnographic Fieldnotes*, 167.

Bibliography

Books, Articles, and Dissertations

Abu-Lughod, Lila. "Writing against Culture." In *Recapturing Anthropology: Working in the Present*, edited by Richard G. Fox, 137–61. Santa Fe, N.M.: School of American Research Press, 1991.

Alpern, Kenneth D., ed. *The Ethics of Reproductive Technology*. New York: Oxford University Press, 1992.

American Society for Reproductive Medicine. Ethics Committee. "Shared-Risk or Refund Programs in Assisted Reproduction." September 1998. <http://www.asrm.org>. Accessed November 2002.

Anderson, Elizabeth. "Is Women's Labor a Commodity?" *Philosophy and Public Affairs* 19, no. 1 (Winter 1990): 71–92.

Andrews, Lori B. *The Clone Age: Adventures in the New World of Reproductive Technology*. New York: Holt, 1999.

———. "My Body, My Property." *Hastings Center Report* 16, no. 5 (October 1986): 28–38.

Arendell, Teresa. *Mothering and Motherhood: A Decade Review*. Working Paper 3. Berkeley: Center for Working Families, University of California, Berkeley, Alfred P. Sloan Center, 1999.

Aronson, Diane. "The Value of a Non-Profit in a Changing World." *RESOLVE National Newsletter* 25, no. 2 (Spring 2000): 2–3.

Bartholet, Elizabeth. *Family Bonds: Adoption and the Politics of Parenting*. Boston: Houghton Mifflin, 1993.

Bazelton, Emily. "See Jane. See Jane Find Another Way. Go Jane." *Washington Post*, May 20, 2001.

Beck, Margaret. "Making the Leap to Adoption." *RESOLVE National Newsletter* 25, no. 4 (Autumn 2000): 1.

Becker, Gay. *The Elusive Embryo: How Women and Men Approach New Reproductive Technologies*. Berkeley: University of California Press, 2000.

Bellah, Robert N., Richard Madsen, William M. Sullivan, Ann Swidler, and Steven M. Tipton. *The Good Society*. New York: Vintage, 1991.

Benhabib, Seyla. *Situating the Self: Gender, Community, and Postmodernism in Contemporary Ethics*. New York: Routledge, 1992.

Benhabib, Seyla, Judith Butler, Drucilla Cornell, and Nancy Fraser. *Feminist Contentions: A Philosophical Exchange*. New York: Routledge, 1995.

Berg, Barbara J. "Listening to the Voices of the Infertile." In *Reproduction, Ethics, and the Law: Feminist Perspectives*, edited by Joan C. Callahan, 80–108. Bloomington: Indiana University Press, 1995.

Berger, Peter. "From the Crisis of Religion to the Crisis of Secularity." In *Religion and America: Spiritual Life in a Secular Age*, edited by Mary Douglas and Steven Tipton, 14–24. Boston: Beacon, 1983.

Bourdieu, Pierre. *Distinction: A Social Critique of the Judgment of Taste*. Cambridge: Harvard University Press, 1984.

Brandeis, Louis, and Samuel Warren. "The Right to Privacy." *Harvard Law Review* 4, no. 5 (December 15, 1890): 193.

Browning, Don S., Bonnie J. Miller-McLemore, Pamela D. Couture, K. Brynolf Lyon, and Robert M. Franklin. *From Culture Wars to Common Ground: Religion and the American Family Debate*. Louisville, Ky.: Westminster John Knox, 1998.

Buber, Martin. *I and Thou*. New York: Scribner's, 1970.

Burawoy, Michael. *Ethnography Unbound: Power and Resistance in the Modern Metropolis*. Berkeley: University of California Press, 1991.

Cahill, Lisa Sowle. "Embodiment and Moral Critique: A Christian Social Perspective." In *Embodiment, Morality, and Medicine*, edited by Lisa Sowle Cahill and Margaret A. Farley, 199–216. Boston: Kluwer Academic, 1995.

——. *Sex, Gender, and Christian Ethics*. Cambridge: Cambridge University Press, 1996.

Centers for Disease Control and Prevention, American Society for Reproductive Medicine, and Society for Assisted Reproductive Technology. "2002 Assisted Reproductive Technology Success Rates: National Summary and Fertility Clinic Reports." December 2004. <http://www.cdc.gov/ART/ART02/PDF/ART2002.pdf>. Accessed March 16, 2007.

Centers for Disease Control and Prevention, American Society for Reproductive Medicine, Society for Assisted Reproductive Technology, and RESOLVE. "1997 Assisted Reproductive Technology Success Rates: National Summary and Fertility Clinic Reports." December 1999. <http://www.cdc.gov/ART/ArchivedART PDFs/97art.pdf>. Accessed March 16, 2007.

——. "1998 Assisted Reproductive Technology Success Rates: National Summary and Fertility Clinic Reports." December 2000. <http://www.cdc.gov/ART/Archived ARTPDFs/art1998.pdf>. Accessed March 16, 2007.

——. "1999 Assisted Reproductive Technology Success Rates: National Summary and

Fertility Clinic Reports." December 2001. <http://www.cdc.gov/ART/Archived ARTPDFs/1999ART_accessible_erat.pdf>. Accessed March 16, 2007.

Chandra, Anjani, and William D. Mosher. "The Demography of Infertility and the Use of Medical Care for Infertility." *Infertility and Reproductive Medicine Clinics of North America* 5, no. 2 (1994): 283–96.

Chandra, Anjani, and Elizabeth Hervey Stephen. "Impaired Fecundity in the United States: 1982–1995." *Family Planning Perspectives* 30, no. 1 (January–February 1998): 34–42.

Clements, Dan. "A Process of Understanding for Men." *RESOLVE of Georgia Newsletter*, Holiday 2000, 6. Reprinted from *Dallas-Fort Worth RESOLVE Newsletter* (1995).

Coleman, John A. "Every Theology Implies a Sociology and Vice Versa." In *Theology and the Social Sciences*, edited by Michael Horace Barnes, 12–33. Maryknoll, N.Y.: Orbis, 2000.

Committee of Inquiry into Human Fertilisation and Embryology. *Report of the Committee of Inquiry into Human Fertilisation and Embryology*. London: Her Majesty's Stationery Office, 1984.

Congregation for the Doctrine of the Faith. "*Donum Vitae*: Instruction on Respect for Human Life in Its Origin and on the Dignity of Procreation" (1987). In *On Moral Medicine: Theological Perspectives in Medical Ethics*, edited by Stephen E. Lammers and Allen Verhey, 469–85. Grand Rapids, Mich.: Eerdmans, 1998.

Connor, Steve. "Frozen Ovary Banks to Offer Childbirth in Later Life." *Independent* (United Kingdom), January 24, 2002.

Cook, Catherine. "Religion and Infertility: Different Views." *RESOLVE of Georgia Newsletter*, Winter 2001, 17–18.

Corea, Gena. *The Mother Machine: Reproductive Technologies from Artificial Insemination to Artificial Wombs*. New York: Harper and Row, 1985.

Corea, Gena, Renate Duelli Klein, Jalna Hanmer, Helen B. Holmes, Betty Hoskins, Madhu Kishwar, Janice Raymond, Robyn Rowland, and Roberta Steinbacher. *Man-Made Women: How New Reproductive Technologies Affect Women*. Bloomington: Indiana University Press, 1987.

Crittenden, Ann. *The Price of Motherhood: Why the Most Important Job in the World Is Still the Least Valued*. New York: Metropolitan, 2001.

Curlin, Farr, and Daniel Hall. "Red Medicine, Blue Medicine: Pluralism and the Future of Healthcare." May 2005. Marty Center Religion and Culture Web Forum, <http://marty-center.uchicago.edu/webforum>. Accessed April 10, 2007.

Curran, Charles E., Margaret A. Farley, and Richard A. McCormick, eds. *Feminist Ethics and the Catholic Moral Tradition*. Readings in Moral Theology 9. New York: Paulist, 1996.

Davis, Dena. "Genetic Dilemmas and the Child's Right to an Open Future." *Hastings Center Report* 27, no. 2 (March–April 1997): 7–15.

DeBaun, M. R., E. L. Niemitz, and A. P. Feinberg. "Association of in Vitro Fertilization with Beckwith-Wiedemann Syndrome and Epigenetic Alterations of LIT1 and H19." *American Journal of Human Genetics* 72, no. 1 (January 2003): 156–60.

Dewey, John. "The Need for a Recovery of Philosophy" (1917). In *The Essential Dewey*. Vol. 1, *Pragmatism, Education, Democracy*, edited by Larry Hickman and Thomas Alexander, 46–70. Bloomington: Indiana University Press, 1998.

Donchin, Anne. "Feminist Critiques of New Fertility Technologies: Implications for Social Policy." *Journal of Medicine and Philosophy* 21, no. 5 (October 1996): 475–98.

———. "The Future of Mothering: Reproductive Technology and Feminist Theory." *Hypatia* 1, no. 2 (Fall 1986): 121–37.

Doyle, Kate. "Advocacy Action." *RESOLVE National Newsletter* 26, no. 2 (Spring 2001): 12.

Dworkin, Ronald. *Life's Dominion: An Argument about Abortion, Euthanasia, and Individual Freedom*. New York: Knopf, 1993.

Eliasoph, Nina. *Avoiding Politics: How Americans Produce Apathy in Everyday Life*. Cambridge: Cambridge University Press, 1998.

Elliot, Carl. *Better Than Well: American Medicine Meets the American Dream*. New York: Norton, 2003.

Elshtain, Jean Bethke. *Public Man, Private Woman: Women in Social and Political Thought*. Princeton: Princeton University Press, 1981.

Emerson, Robert, Rachel Fretz, and Linda Shaw. *Writing Ethnographic Fieldnotes*. Chicago: University of Chicago Press, 1995.

Engelhardt, H. Tristram, Jr. *The Foundations of Bioethics*. New York: Oxford University Press, 1996.

Farley, Margaret A. "Feminist Ethics." In *The Westminster Dictionary of Christian Ethics*, edited by James F. Childress and John Macquarrie, 229–31. Philadelphia: Westminster, 1986.

———. "Feminist Theology and Bioethics." In *On Moral Medicine: Theological Perspectives in Medical Ethics*, edited by Stephen E. Lammers and Allen Verhey, 90–103. Grand Rapids, Mich.: Eerdmans, 1998.

Firestone, Shulamith. *The Dialectic of Sex*. New York: Bantam, 1970.

Flyvbjerg, Bent. *Making Social Science Matter: Why Social Inquiry Fails and How It Can Succeed Again*. Cambridge: Cambridge University Press, 2001.

Folbre, Nancy. *The Invisible Heart: Economics and Family Values*. New York: New Press, 2001.

Fraser, Nancy. "Rethinking the Public Sphere." In *Justice Interruptus: Critical Reflections on the "Postsocialist" Condition*, 69–98. New York: Routledge, 1997.

Gerson, Kathleen. *No Man's Land: Men's Changing Commitments to Family and Work*. New York: Basic, 1993.

Ginsberg, Faye, and Rayna Rapp, eds. *Conceiving the New World Order: The Global Politics of Reproduction*. Berkeley: University of California Press, 1995.

Glendon, Mary Ann. "Is the Economic Emancipation of Women Today Contrary to a Healthy, Functioning Family?" In *The Family, Civil Society, and the State*, edited by Christopher Wolfe, 87–95. Lanham, Md.: Rowman and Littlefield, 1998.

——. *Rights Talk: The Impoverishment of Political Discourse*. New York: Free Press, 1991.

Goodman, Ellen. "Overwork Overwhelms Families of the 90s." *Boston Globe*, October 6, 1994.

Greil, Arthur. *Not Yet Pregnant: Infertile Couples in Contemporary America*. New Brunswick, N.J.: Rutgers University Press, 1991.

Gudorf, Christine. "Parenting, Mutual Love, and Sacrifice." In *Women's Consciousness, Women's Conscience*, edited by Barbara Hilkert Andolsen, Christine E. Gudorf, and Mary D. Pellauer, 175–91. Minneapolis, Minn.: Winston, 1985.

Gustafson, James. *Intersections: Science, Theology, and Ethics*. Cleveland: Pilgrim, 1996.

Habermas, Jürgen. *Moral Consciousness and Communicative Action*. Cambridge: MIT Press, 1990.

——. *The Structural Transformation of the Public Sphere: An Inquiry into a Category of Bourgeois Society*. Cambridge: MIT Press, 1989.

Hays, Sharon. *The Cultural Contradictions of Motherhood*. New Haven: Yale University Press, 1996.

Heatherley, Joyce Landorf. *Balcony People*. Salado, Tex.: Balcony, 1989.

Hewlett, Sylvia Ann. *Creating a Life: Professional Women and the Quest for Children*. New York: Talk Miramax, 2002.

Hidlebaugh, D. A., I. E. Thompson, and M. J. Berger. "Cost of Assisted Reproductive Technologies for a Health Maintenance Organization." *Journal of Reproductive Medicine* 42, no. 9 (September 1997): 570–74.

Hochman, Anndee. *Everyday Acts and Small Subversions: Women Reinventing Family, Community, and Home*. Portland, Ore.: Eighth Mountain, 1994.

Hochschild, Arlie Russell. *The Second Shift*. New York: Avon, 1989.

——. *The Time Bind: When Work Becomes Home and Home Becomes Work*. New York: Metropolitan, 1997.

Hodder, Harbour Fraser. "The New Fertility: The Promise—and Perils—of Human Reproductive Technologies." *Harvard Magazine*, November–December 1997, 54–64, 97–99.

Holland, Suzanne. "Contested Commodities at Both Ends of Life: Buying and Selling Gametes, Embryos, and Body Tissues." *Kennedy Institute of Ethics Journal* 11, no. 3 (September 2001): 263–84.

Inhorn, Marcia. *Local Babies, Global Science: Gender, Religion, and in Vitro Fertilization in Egypt*. New York: Routledge, 2003.

Institute for Reproductive Medicine at Saint Barnabas Medical Center, "Statement in Regard to Cytoplasmic Transfer." May 18, 2001. <http://infertility.about.com>. Accessed November 2002.

Jacobs, Jerry, and Kathleen Gerson. "Who Are the Overworked Americans?" *Review of Social Economy* 56, no. 4 (Winter 1998): 442–59.

Jonsen, Albert. "Theological Ethics, Bioethics, and Public Moral Discourse." *Kennedy Institute of Ethics Journal* 4, no. 1 (March 1994): 1–12.

Kalb, Claudia. "The Truth about Fertility: Why Doctors Are Warning That Science Can't Beat the Biological Clock." *Newsweek*, August 13, 2001, 40–49.

Keller, Larry. "Dual Earners: Double Trouble." November 13, 2000. <http://archives.cnn.com/2000/CAREER/trends/11/13/dual.earners/index.html>. Accessed March 16, 2007.

Kittay, Eva Feder. *Love's Labor: Essays on Women, Equality, and Dependency*. New York: Routledge, 1999.

Kolata, Gina. "Fertility, Inc.: Clinics Race to Lure Clients." *New York Times*, January 1, 2002.

Kübler-Ross, Elisabeth. *On Death and Dying*. New York: Macmillan, 1969.

Kurzman, Charles. "Convincing Sociologists: Values and Interests in the Sociology of Knowledge." In *Ethnography Unbound: Power and Resistance in the Modern Metropolis*, edited by Michael Burawoy, 250–70. Berkeley: University of California Press, 1991.

Lasker, Judith, and Susan Borg. *In Search of Parenthood*. Boston: Beacon, 1987.

Lebacqz, Karen. "Diversity, Disability, and Designer Genes: On What It Means to Be Human." *Studia Theologica* 50, no. 1 (1996): 3–14.

Madsen, Richard, William Sullivan, Ann Swidler, and Steven Tipton. *Meaning and Modernity: Religion, Polity, and Self*. Berkeley: University of California Press, 2001.

Margolis, Diane. *The Fabric of Self: A Theory of Ethics and Emotions*. New Haven: Yale University Press, 1998.

Martin, Emily. *The Woman in the Body: A Cultural Analysis of Reproduction*. Boston: Beacon, 1987.

Massey, Joe B. "Low Ovarian Reserve: The Silent Cause of Infertility in the Modern Era." *RESOLVE of Georgia Newsletter*, Holiday 2000, 1.

May, Elaine Tyler. *Barren in the Promised Land: Childless Americans and the Pursuit of Happiness*. New York: Basic, 1995.

Mead, Rebecca. "Eggs for Sale." *New Yorker*, August 9, 1999, 56–65.

Meilaender, Gilbert. *Body, Soul, and Bioethics*. Notre Dame, Ind.: University of Notre Dame Press, 1995.

——. "A Child of One's Own: At What Price?" In *The Reproduction Revolution: A Christian Appraisal of Sexuality, Reproductive Technologies, and the Family*, edited by John F. Kilner, Paige C. Cunningham, and W. David Hager, 36–45. Grand Rapids, Mich.: Eerdmans, 2000.

Meyer, John W. "Self and Life Course: Institutionalization and Its Effects." In *Institutional Structures*, edited by G. M. Thomas, J. W. Meyer, F. O. Ramirez, and J. Boli, 242–60. London: Sage, 1987.

Mill, John Stuart. "On Liberty" (1859). In *On Liberty and Other Writings*, edited by Stefan Collini, 1–115. Cambridge: Cambridge University Press, 1989.

Miller-McLemore, Bonnie J. *Also a Mother: Work and Family as Theological Dilemma*. Nashville, Tenn.: Abingdon, 1994.

——. "Produce or Perish: Generativity and New Reproductive Technologies." *Journal of the American Academy of Religion* 59, no. 1 (Spring 1991): 39–69.

Mitchie, Helena, and Naomi Cahn. *Confinements: Fertility and Infertility in Contemporary Culture*. New Brunswick, N.J.: Rutgers University Press, 1997.

Morgen, Sandra. *Into Our Own Hands: The Women's Health Movement in the United States, 1969–1990*. New Brunswick, N.J.: Rutgers University Press, 2002.

Murphy, Julien. "Should Lesbians Count as Infertile Couples? Antilesbian Discrimination in Assisted Reproduction." In *Embodying Bioethics: Recent Feminist Advances*, edited by Anne Donchin and Laura Purdy, 103–20. Lanham, Md.: Rowman and Littlefield, 1999.

National Partnership for Women and Families. *Guide to the Family and Medical Leave Act: Questions and Answers*. 4th ed. Washington, D.C.: National Partnership for Women and Families, 1998.

Neumann, Peter J., S. D. Gharib, and M. C. Weinstein. "The Cost of a Successful Delivery with in Vitro Fertilization." *New England Journal of Medicine* 331, no. 4 (July 28, 1994): 239–43.

Niebuhr, H. Richard. *The Responsible Self: An Essay in Christian Moral Philosophy*. New York: Harper and Row, 1963.

Nussbaum, Martha C. *Sex and Social Justice*. New York: Oxford University Press, 1999.

O'Connor, Anahad. "U.S. Infant Mortality Rate Rises Slightly." *New York Times*, February 12, 2004.

O'Donovan, Oliver. *Begotten or Made?* Oxford: Clarendon, 1984.

Okin, Susan Moller. *Justice, Gender, and the Family*. New York: Basic, 1989.

Pappert, Ann. "A Special Report on the Fertility Industry: What Price Pregnancy?" *Ms.*, June–July 2000, 43–49.

Parens, Erik. "The Goodness of Fragility: On the Prospect of Genetic Technologies Aimed at the Enhancement of Human Capacities." *Kennedy Institute of Ethics Journal* 5, no. 2 (June 1995): 141–53.

Paul VI. *Humanae Vitae: Encyclical Letter of His Holiness on the Regulation of Birth* (1968). In *On Moral Medicine: Theological Perspectives in Medical Ethics*, edited by Stephen E. Lammers and Allen Verhey, 434–38. Grand Rapids, Mich.: Eerdmans, 1998.

Pollitt, Katha. "Backlash Babies." *The Nation*, May 13, 2002. <http://www.thenation.com>. Accessed May 14, 2002.

President's Council on Bioethics. *Reproduction and Responsibility: The Regulation of New Biotechnologies*. Washington, D.C.: President's Council on Bioethics, 2004.

Radin, Margaret Jane. *Contested Commodities: The Trouble with Trade in Sex, Children, Body Parts, and Other Things*. Cambridge: Harvard University Press, 1996.

Rapp, Rayna. *Testing Women, Testing the Fetus: The Social Impact of Amniocentesis in America*. New York: Routledge, 1999.

Rausch, Diedre. "Trust: A Vital Component of the Infertility Journey." *RESOLVE National Newsletter* 25, no. 3 (Summer 2000): 1.

Rawls, John. *Political Liberalism*. New York: Columbia University Press, 1996.

——. *A Theory of Justice*. Cambridge: Harvard University Press, 1971.

Raymond, Janice. *Women as Wombs: Reproductive Technologies and the Battle over Women's Freedom*. San Francisco: HarperCollins, 1993.

Reich, Warren Thomas. "Speaking of Suffering: A Moral Account of Compassion." *Soundings* 72, no. 1 (Spring 1989): 83–108.

RESOLVE. *Fact Sheet: Donor Egg*. Fact sheet 24. Somerville, Mass.: RESOLVE, 1999.

——. *Infertility and Insurance Coverage: A Briefing Paper*. Somerville, Mass.: RESOLVE, n.d.

——. *Managing Family and Friends*. Somerville, Mass.: RESOLVE, n.d.

——. "Overview of the CDC's Model Certification Program for Embryo Laboratories." <www.resolve.org>. Accessed August 2001.

——. *When You're Wishing for a Baby: Myths and Facts*. Somerville, Mass.: RESOLVE, n.d.

RESOLVE and the National Endowment for Financial Education. *Planning to Afford Family Building: Financial Planning and Infertility*. Somerville, Mass.: RESOLVE, 1999.

RESOLVE and the National Partnership for Women and Families. *Infertility and Adoption: How the FMLA Can Help*. Washington, D.C.: National Partnership for Women and Families, 1998.

RESOLVE, with Diane Aronson. *Resolving Infertility: Understanding the Options and Choosing Solutions When You Want to Have a Baby*. New York: HarperCollins, 1999.

Risman, Barbara J. *Gender Vertigo: American Families in Transition*. New Haven: Yale University Press, 1998.

Roberts, Dorothy. *Killing the Black Body: Race, Reproduction, and the Meaning of Liberty*. New York: Pantheon, 1997.

Robertson, John. *Children of Choice: Freedom and the New Reproductive Technologies*. Princeton: Princeton University Press, 1994.

Rosen, Christine. *Preaching Eugenics: Religious Leaders and the American Eugenics Movement*. New York: Oxford University Press, 2004.

Rosenblatt, Roger, ed. *Consuming Desires: Consumption, Culture, and the Pursuit of Happiness*. Washington, D.C.: Island, 1999.

Rothman, Barbara Katz. *Recreating Motherhood: Ideology and Technology in a Patriarchal Society*. New York: Norton, 1989.

Rowland, Robyn. *Living Laboratories: Women and Reproductive Technologies*. Bloomington: Indiana University Press, 1992.

Ruzek, Sheryl. "The History and Future of Women's Health." June 11, 1998. Seminar sponsored by the Office on Women's Health and PHS Coordinating Committee on Women's Health, <http://www.4woman.gov/owh/pub/history/healthmvmt.htm>.Accessed June 2, 2005.

Ryan, Maura. "The Argument for Unlimited Procreative Liberty: A Feminist Critique." In *Feminist Ethics and the Catholic Moral Tradition*, edited by C. E. Curran, M. A. Farley, R. A. McCormick, 383–401. New York: Paulist, 1996.

——. "Justice and Artificial Reproduction: A Catholic Feminist Analysis." Ph.D. diss., Yale University, 1993.

Sandelowski, Margarete, and Sheryl de Lacy. "The Uses of a 'Disease': Infertility as Rhetorical Vehicle." In *Infertility around the Globe: New Thinking on Childlessness, Gender, and Reproductive Technologies*, edited by Marcia Inhorn and Frank van Balen, 33–51. Berkeley: University of California Press, 2002.

Sandel, Michael. "The Case against Perfection." *Atlantic Monthly*, April 2004, 50–62.

Schor, Juliet B. *The Overworked American: The Unexpected Decline of Leisure*. New York: Basic, 1992.

——. "What's Wrong with Consumer Society?: Competitive Spending and the 'New Consumerism.'" In *Consuming Desires: Consumption, Culture, and the Pursuit of Happiness*, edited by Roger Rosenblatt, 37–50. Washington, D.C.: Island, 1999.

"Scientists Manufacture Human Eggs." *Washington Post*, July 2, 2001. <http://www.washingtonpost.com>. Accessed July 3, 2001.

Serono. *Infertility: The Emotional Roller Coaster* (patient education booklet). Norwell, Mass.: Serono Laboratories, 1997.

Sherwin, Susan. *No Longer Patient: Feminist Ethics and Health Care*. Philadelphia: Temple University Press, 1992.

Shklar, Judith. *The Faces of Injustice*. New Haven: Yale University Press, 1990.

Soelle, Dorothee. *Suffering*. Philadelphia: Fortress, 1975.

Spain, Daphne, and Suzanne Bianchi. *Balancing Act: Motherhood, Marriage, and Employment among American Women*. New York: Sage, 1996.

Spallone, Patricia. *Beyond Conception: The New Politics of Reproduction*. Granby, Mass.: Bergin and Garvey, 1989.

Spar, Deborah. *The Baby Business: How Money, Science, and Politics Drive the Commerce of Conception*. Boston: Harvard Business School Press, 2006.

Spradley, James P. *The Ethnographic Interview*. New York: Holt, Rinehart, and Winston, 1979.

Stanworth, Michelle, ed. *Reproductive Technologies: Gender, Motherhood, and Medicine*. Minneapolis: University of Minnesota Press, 1987.

Starr, Paul. *The Social Transformation of American Medicine*. New York: HarperCollins, 1982.

Stephen, Elizabeth Hervey. "Projections of Impaired Fecundity among Women in the United States: 1995–2020." *Fertility and Sterility* 66, no. 2 (August 1996): 205–9.

Stephen, Elizabeth Hervey, and Anjani Chandra. "Use of Infertility Services in the United States: 1995." *Family Planning Perspectives* 32, no. 3 (May–June 2000): 132–37.

Stock, Gregory. "Eggs for Sale: How Much Is Too Much?" *American Journal of Bioethics* 1, no. 4 (Fall 2001): 26–27.

Stolberg, Sheryl Gay. "Buying Years for Women on the Biological Clock." *New York Times*, October 3, 1999.

Swidler, Ann. "In Groups We Trust." Review of *Sharing the Journey: Support Groups and America's New Quest for Community*, by Robert Wuthnow. *New York Times Book Review*, March 20, 1994.

Taylor, Janelle. "An All-Consuming Experience: Obstetrical Ultrasound and the Commodification of Pregnancy." In *Biotechnology and Culture: Bodies, Anxieties, Ethics*, edited by Paul E. Browdin, 147–70. Bloomington: Indiana University Press, 2000.

Thomasma, David. "Selling Human Egg Donation." *American Journal of Bioethics* 1, no. 4 (Fall 2001): 28.

Thompson, Charis M. "Fertile Ground: Feminists Theorize Infertility." In *Infertility around the Globe: New Thinking on Childlessness, Gender, and Reproductive Technologies*, edited by Marcia C. Inhorn and Frank van Balen, 52–78. Berkeley: University of California Press, 2002.

Toner, Jim. "Your Medical Questions Answered." *RESOLVE National Newsletter* 26, no. 1 (Winter 2001): 1–7.

Tong, Rosemarie. "Feminist Approaches to Bioethics." In *Feminism and Bioethics: Beyond Reproduction*, edited by Susan M. Wolf, 67–94. New York: Oxford University Press, 1996.

Tucker, Michael. "Freezing Human Eggs." *RESOLVE of Georgia Newsletter*, Summer 2000, 1.

U.S. Congress, Office of Technology Assessment. *Infertility: Medical and Social Choices*. OTA-BA-358. Washington, D.C.: U.S. Government Printing Office, 1988.

Vallis, Mary. "McGill Pill Could Reshape Fertility: Early-Stage Research: Intent Is to Enable Women to Hoard Eggs for Later Years." *National Post* (Canada), July 20, 2000. <http://www.canada.com/nationalpost/index.html>. Accessed July 21, 2000.

van Balen, Frank. "The Psychologization of Infertility." In *Infertility around the Globe: New Thinking on Childlessness, Gender, and Reproductive Technologies*, edited by Marcia C. Inhorn and Frank van Balen, 79–98. Berkeley: University of California Press, 2002.

Volf, Miroslav. "The Gift of Infertility." *Christian Century*, June 14, 2005, 33.

Walzer, Michael. *Spheres of Justice*. New York: Basic, 1983.

Weber, Max. *The Protestant Ethic and the Spirit of Capitalism*. Los Angeles: Roxbury, 1998.

——. "Science as a Vocation." In *From Max Weber: Essays in Sociology*, edited by H. H. Gerth and C. Wright Mills, 129–56. New York: Oxford University Press, 1958.

Weil, Elizabeth. "A Wrongful Birth?" *New York Times Magazine*, March 12, 2006.

Weschler, Toni. *Taking Charge of Your Fertility: The Definitive Guide to Natural Birth Control and Pregnancy Achievement*. New York: HarperCollins, 1995.

Wilcox, Lynne S., and William D. Mosher. "Use of Infertility Services in the United States." *Obstetrics and Gynecology* 82, no. 1 (July 1993): 122–27.

Wolf, Susan. "Pre-Implantation Genetic Diagnosis and the Ethics of 'Creating Donors.'" Paper presented at the American Society of Bioethics and Humanities annual meeting, Nashville, Tenn., October 25, 2001.

Woliver, Laura R. "The Deflective Power of Reproductive Technologies: The Impact on Women." *Women and Politics* 9, no. 3 (1989): 17–47.

——. "Reproductive Technologies, Surrogacy Arrangements, and the Politics of Motherhood." In *Mothers in Law: Feminist Theory and the Legal Regulation of Motherhood*, edited by Martha Albertson Fineman and Isabel Karpin, 346–59. New York: Columbia University Press, 1995.

Wuthnow, Robert. *Sharing the Journey: Support Groups and America's New Quest for Community*. New York: Free Press, 1994.

Young, Iris Marion. *Intersecting Voices: Dilemmas of Gender, Political Philosophy, and Policy*. Princeton: Princeton University Press, 1997.

Internet Sources

American Society for Reproductive Medicine. <http://www.asrm.org>. Accessed June 2005.

Center for Drug Evaluation and Research, New and Generic Drug Approvals: 1998–2004. <http://www.fda.gov/cder/approval/index.htm>. Accessed June 23, 2005.

Child Welfare Information Gateway. <http://www.childwelfare.gov>. Accessed April 10, 2007.

Extend Fertility. <http://www.extendfertility.com>. Accessed April 12, 2007.

Georgia Chapter, RESOLVE: The National Infertility Organization. <http://www.resolveofgeorgia.org>. Accessed April 10, 2007.

Georgia Reproductive Specialists. <http://www.ivf.com>. Accessed January 10, 2001.

The President's Council on Bioethics. <http://www.bioethics.gov>. Accessed April 10, 2007.

RESOLVE: The National Infertility Organization. <http://www.resolve.org>. Accessed March 15, 2000.

RESOLVE Corporate Council. <http://www.resolve.org/site/PageServer?pagename=cpsp_home>. Accessed April 10, 2007.

U.S. Department of Health and Human Services, Centers for Disease Control and

Prevention, National Center for Health Statistics/National Survey of Family
Growth. <http://www.cdc.gov/nchs/nsfg>. Accessed 2002.

U.S. Department of Health and Human Services, Centers for Disease Control and
Prevention, Reproductive Health: Home. <http://www.cdc.gov/reproductive
health/index.htm>. Accessed April 10, 2007.

Xytex Sperm Bank. <http://www.xytex.com>. Accessed April 10, 2007.

Index

Abortion, 27, 28, 54, 158, 161, 180 (n. 23), 196 (n. 55), 200 (n. 4)

Abu-Lughod, Lila, 6

Adoption, 2, 27, 39, 44, 46, 47, 49, 51, 52, 55, 56, 57, 65, 66, 72, 76, 77, 85, 86, 95, 96, 97, 102, 118, 124, 133, 134, 138, 140, 142–43, 150, 151, 152, 154, 157, 163, 164, 168, 169, 184 (n. 88), 190 (nn. 70, 71), 199 (n. 39); compared with ART, 71, 194 (n. 35); compared with gamete donation, 34, 87, 94, 95, 148, 150, 184 (n. 89); costs of, 76, 81, 189 (n. 55); and race, 80–82, 112; RESOLVE annual symposium on, 39–40, 47, 70, 75, 76, 82, 171; special-needs adoption, 80–81, 82

Advanced reproductive technologies, 39. *See also* Assisted reproductive technologies

American College of Obstetricians and Gynecologists, 43

American Society of Reproductive Medicine (ASRM), 5, 13, 42, 43, 45, 50, 171, 178 (n. 9)

Americans with Disabilities Act, 43

Aquinas, Thomas, 121

Aristotle, 121, 195 (n. 53)

Aronson, Diane, 50

Artificial insemination, 10, 11, 26, 27, 42, 134, 152, 196 (n. 55). *See also* Intrauterine insemination

Assisted reproductive technologies (ART), 10–12, 17, 22, 32, 33, 45, 47, 110, 127, 177 (n. 3), 182 (n. 65), 198 (n. 14); as consumer item, 77, 79, 80, 87, 98, 101, 113, 130, 157; costs of, 13–14, 76–77, 113, 149, 185 (n. 11); cytoplasmic transfer, 12, 100, 120, 196 (n. 62); decision-making factors in, 6, 7, 70, 76, 81, 89, 96, 97, 105, 107, 116, 122–24, 132, 133, 138, 151, 158, 164, 173, 178 (n. 15), 196 (n. 62); and delayed childbearing, 4, 20, 99, 101, 105, 138, 167, 168, 173, 178 (n. 7); demographics of use of, 4, 5, 12–13, 15, 40, 76, 110–13, 135; ethical issues in, 2, 5–6, 8, 9, 15–16, 21, 23, 26, 36, 45, 56, 84, 86, 100, 107, 109, 112, 115, 124, 130, 133, 134, 136–37, 147, 149, 151, 154, 160, 161, 164, 172, 173, 183 (nn. 76, 78), 194 (n. 89); gamete intrafallopian transfer (GIFT), 10, 11, 179 (n. 2); gender issues in, 8, 24, 73, 98, 102, 103, 104, 105, 171; goals of use of, 5, 16, 18, 25, 56, 99, 114, 117, 121, 122, 131, 137, 142, 151, 158, 160, 167, 168, 177 (n. 7); health risks of, 3, 5, 7, 20–21, 35–36, 44–46, 100, 120, 126,

Suffering, 55, 59, 65, 66, 118, 132, 139, 141, 145, 146, 147, 148, 165, 198 (n. 29)

Superovulation, 11

Support group, 48, 58

Surrogacy, 11, 17, 27, 30, 47, 49, 87, 88, 99, 138, 169, 184 (n. 86), 186 (n. 31), 193 (n. 1), 196 (n. 55), 199 (n. 64)

Swidler, Ann, 58

Swift, Jane, 182 (n. 46)

Technological imperative, 194 (n. 35)

Therapists: as speakers at RESOLVE, 46, 47, 48, 59, 68–69, 71, 72, 75, 76, 85, 86, 102, 104, 109, 134, 135, 139, 147, 158, 168, 171, 173, 186 (n. 31), 188 (n. 7), 192 (n. 115), 195 (n. 38)

Therapy, 77, 90, 146, 147, 148

Third-party gamete donation, 30, 31, 32, 33–34, 35, 37, 47, 87, 92, 93, 94, 95, 96, 138, 150–65 passim, 169, 184 (n. 86), 190 (n. 71), 193 (n. 1), 199 (n. 64); versus adoption, 94, 148, 150; and analogy with blood donation, 94, 154, 155; and issues of stigma, 92, 95, 96; and matching for race, 81, 97; regulation of, 44, 45. *See also* Egg donation

Transformation, 40. *See also* Infertility

United Kingdom: approach to regulating ART, 128; first successful IVF in, 10; Human Fertilisation and Embryology Authority (HFEA), 127, 128

United States: and American eugenics movement, 162; approach to regulating ART, 45, 127–29, 157, 159; fertil-ity clinics in, 12, 179 (n. 9); Fertility Clinic Success Rate and Certification Act of 1992, 14, 129; first use of ART in, 21, 182 (n. 47); regional differences in ART use in, 145, 161; total spent on infertility treatments in, 43

United States Supreme Court, 123. *See also* Legal decisions

Universalizable norms, 32–33, 34, 183 (n. 83)

Vatican, 30, 33

Volunteerism, 90, 91, 105, 106, 116, 117

Weber, Max, 119, 195 (n. 48)

"Welcome to Holland" parable, 141–42, 146, 198 (n. 31)

Wolf, Susan, 123, 196 (n. 62)

Woliver, Laura, 25, 107

Women's health movement, 53

Work and family, 2, 3, 7, 8, 35, 36, 66–67, 75, 103, 105–9, 117, 132; and care for dependents, 4, 19, 102, 103, 108, 193 (n. 11), 196 (n. 59); changes in U.S. work, 19; conflicts between, 5, 6, 7, 9, 26, 87, 105, 164, 173; differences according to class, 19–20, 181 (n. 38); differences according to race, 19, 181 (n. 38); and DINKs, 76; and gender, 4, 8, 19–20, 73, 89, 90, 103, 104; and overwork, 19–20, 87, 109, 114

Wrongful life, 123

Wuthnow, Robert, 58–59, 60, 61

Xytex, 193 (n. 1)

Young, Iris Marion, 151

Studies in Social Medicine

Nancy M. P. King, Gail E. Henderson, and Jane Stein, eds., *Beyond Regulations: Ethics in Human Subjects Research* (1999).

Laurie Zoloth, *Health Care and the Ethics of Encounter: A Jewish Discussion of Social Justice* (1999).

Susan M. Reverby, ed., *Tuskegee's Truths: Rethinking the Tuskegee Syphilis Study* (2000).

Beatrix Hoffman, *The Wages of Sickness: The Politics of Health Insurance in Progressive America* (2000).

Margarete Sandelowski, *Devices and Desires: Gender, Technology, and American Nursing* (2000).

Keith Wailoo, *Dying in the City of the Blues: Sickle Cell Anemia and the Politics of Race and Health* (2001).

Judith Andre, *Bioethics as Practice* (2002).

Chris Feudtner, *Bittersweet: Diabetes, Insulin, and the Transformation of Illness* (2003).

Ann Folwell Stanford, *Bodies in a Broken World: Women Novelists of Color and the Politics of Medicine* (2003).

Lawrence O. Gostin, *The AIDS Pandemic: Complacency, Injustice, and Unfulfilled Expectations* (2004).

Arthur A. Daemmrich, *Pharmacopolitics: Drug Regulation in the United States and Germany* (2004).

Carl Elliott and Tod Chambers, eds., *Prozac as a Way of Life* (2004).

Steven M. Stowe, *Doctoring the South: Southern Physicians and Everyday Medicine in the Mid–Nineteenth Century* (2004).

Arleen Marcia Tuchman, *Science Has No Sex: The Life of Marie Zakrzewska, M.D.* (2006).

Michael H. Cohen, *Healing at the Borderland of Medicine and Religion* (2006).

Keith Wailoo, Julie Livingston, and Peter Guarnaccia, eds., *A Death Retold: Jesica Santillan, the Bungled Transplant, and Paradoxes of Medical Citizenship* (2006).

Michelle T. Moran, *Colonizing Leprosy: Imperialism and the Politics of Public Health in the United States* (2007).

Karey Harwood, *The Infertility Treadmill: Feminist Ethics, Personal Choice, and the Use of Reproductive Technologies* (2007).